Peptides Made Simple

Usage, Benefits, Dosing, Cycling & More

Matthew Farrahi

Contents

Author's Introduction

In the modern world, many societies have long followed the "sick care" model. It is said that allopathic medicine has repeatedly failed people, ultimately leaving them in a worse spot than they started. The allopathic model focuses on treating symptoms rather than the root cause. To make matters worse, many companies that control the pharmaceutical industry have been doing their due diligence to cover up ways that will sustainably help people on a deeper level.

Why?

Because they will lose profit and ultimately lose control over people. They are scared of what may happen if people can empower themselves and tap into the incredible power we all have inside of us.

The revolution of peptide anecdotes is trying to prove that it can solve the root causes of illness and disease, offer the ability to treat the illness and enhance the body's natural regenerative properties.

Well, my own experience strongly supports that view. I have experienced peptides working with the body to encourage and rapidly accelerate its healing process. Once peptides are used with a healthy and optimized lifestyle, they become the "magic solution" I have been searching for.

How these compounds can be applied are endless. This is one of the many reasons why peptides are so popular. Almost anyone can benefit from peptides.

This book will try to explain

- What peptides are

- What I did not do (the mistakes I avoided that kept me safe)

- An overview of all the most common peptides in the field (how they work, my insights on dosing and cycling, benefits, side effects, etc.)

- The best way I started with peptides in the most efficient and effective manner

- And much more

When I decided it was time for a significant change and embraced the latest in regenerative medicine, I found a new way to take control of my life. Now, I'm excited to share my journey with you.

Notes From the Author

Thank you for purchasing this book and exploring my other informative resources.

This book is a personal account of my exploration into peptides and their potential to enhance various facets of life, all in pursuit of living the fullest. I'm sharing such a journey and experience, hoping it may benefit your life as it did for me.

If you want extensive justification of my views through published or peer-reviewed research, this book might not meet your expectations. I am skeptical of the current state of research. There are instances where study designs may be influenced to attain particular outcomes, and replicability is sometimes a concern.

Based on my observations, I've noticed cases where research is sponsored to further a specific corporate agenda. Additionally, complex medical terminology can sometimes make these studies challenging to understand.

Besides all of this, there is still some truth to research. While exploring peptides, I've encountered various research studies, some offering valuable insights. I've included references to multiple studies in this book for curious people who want to delve deeper. However, I've taken the time to summarize the key points from these studies to provide you with a concise and understandable overview based on my understanding and interpretation.

Matthew's Personal Insight on Dosing and Cycling Schemes in the book comes from reading and studying some of the most renounced clinicians specializing in peptide therapy, from numerous subjective experiences of bio-hackers, and from my own experience with peptides. Anyone researching peptide dosing and cycling schemes finds it difficult to find a common trend. I tried to find a happy medium between all the different perspectives, focusing on the more conservative approach.

But why is it hard to find a peptide's absolute dosing and cycling protocol?

There are a lot of reasons for this.

1. Peptides are an up-and-coming field of regenerative medicine. New information is being discovered every day.

2. Every health practitioner has a different perspective on the best use of the peptide.

3. Depending on the intention of how the peptide is used and whom it's for, it will change the dosing and cycling.

4. Peptides, for the most part, have a high safety profile, giving them a large room to play around and experiment with

5. I've noticed that reactions can vary significantly from person to person. What might require a larger dose for me could potentially need a smaller amount for someone else to experience similar effects. That's why I've learned to be attentive to my body's responses and adjust accordingly.

Finally, I've written this book based on my experiences and extensive exploration of the world of peptides, aiming to share the insights and knowledge I've gathered. However, I'm always on a journey of learning and discovery, finding new pieces of information and understanding. I invite you to do the same and use this book as a starting point and a companion to learning more about peptides. Remember, there's always more to learn and discover, so keep an open mind, continue your research, and, most importantly, listen to your intuition as you navigate this journey.

Disclaimer

The content of this book and any associated materials has not been evaluated, reviewed, assessed, or approved by the Food and Drug Administration or any other medical authority. I do not possess a medical or equivalent degree or professional accreditation, and I intend not to offer any medical advice, opinion, diagnoses, treatments, cures, or prevention strategies for diseases, health, or other related conditions.

The insights and information presented in this book and any associated materials are solely and exclusively based on my personal experiences and other publicly accessible research materials. They should be considered personal opinions and provided solely for the intended purpose. This content is not a substitute or alternative for professional medical advice, opinion, or consultation.

I strongly encourage and recommend that readers independently seek advice/opinion from a qualified healthcare professional/doctor if they wish to apply any of the practices or information found in this book or in any other relevant materials. This is particularly crucial for individuals who are pregnant, nursing, on medication, or dealing with other medical conditions, but it applies to all readers without any limitation.

By engaging with the content of this book, you acknowledge and agree that you are solely responsible for any actions or inactions taken based on the information provided and that the author or publisher is not responsible.

How To Use This Book

I've waded through countless peptide resources and noticed that most are steeped in complex details and medical terms, making it challenging to grasp and use the information. Thus, I've drafted this book through my journey and understanding, aiming to offer you a clear and concise overview of peptides to make the topic straightforward and accessible to all readers.

You may have heard of some or none of the peptides in this book. It is designed to be pulled out to find the peptide or peptide combo that a person may want to learn more about or for a quick refresher.

I recommend starting by reading Peptide 101 all the way through and then choosing a category of peptides to study or a peptide that interests you to read about.

Part 9 of the book switches over to discussing peptide combos. I recommend reading that section thoroughly to understand how I combined peptides safely and efficiently. Parts 10 to 16 focus on several unique peptide combos I crafted.

In the peptide combo section, several parts of different combos are repeated. The peptide combo sections are not designed to be read straight through; instead, they are designed to find a specific combo and understand all its significant aspects.

Part 17 - Starting Your Peptide Research Lab - is excellent for peptide researchers or readers interested in learning more about it. I recommend reading this section all the way through if this interests you.

I will dive deep into all the tools and resources I gathered to create and utilize my peptide research lab. Through trial and error, I've distilled my knowledge of various peptides and their combinations into this book, aiming to present it easily to the reader. My goal is to save you from the endless hours I spent navigating through research and hunting for crucial details, allowing you to gain as much knowledge as possible without feeling lost between scattered information all over the internet.

1. Peptide 101

Why Peptides?

- Peptides work through an endogenous process (naturally occurring). They work with the body.

- Peptides are selective, meaning we can target pathways of the body to heal ourselves faster, optimize our hormones, increase our immune system, etc.

- Peptides offer a lot of potential in helping with metabolic disease and oncology (cancer treatments)

- Embracing peptides has opened my eyes to the empowering potential of managing regenerative treatments from the comfort of my own home, democratizing access to these advanced healing practices.

What Are Peptides?

- There are over 7,000 naturally occurring peptides in the body

- Peptides are molecules that are a combination of two or more amino acids joined together through a peptide bond

- Peptides started getting used in medicine in the 1920's (insulin being the first peptide on the market)

- There are over 150 peptides involved in medical treatments, and over 500 are being studied for future therapeutic use.

- Some peptides work better on your skin, injected under the skin, in the muscle, taken orally, etc. Most commonly, peptides are injected.

How Do Peptides Work?

- Most humans begin to cease making enough signaling agents (peptides) by around age 30

- They exist in all cells.

- Peptides work through an endogenous process (naturally occurring). They work with the body.

- They can function as a messenger for cells to turn different body aspects on and off.

- Most peptides have a short half-life. Signaled → Do their job → Exit. Some peptides are being made to have a longer half-life to increase their effects.

Are Peptides Safe?

My Insights On Safe Peptide Practices

- Practicing proper injecting techniques

- Avoiding peptide misuse

- Selecting the appropriate peptides

I have cultivated a unique perspective and experience. I have termed this Matthew's Personal Insight on Dosing, a resource that I trust will be valuable to readers and researchers, contributing to safer peptide practices for all involved.

My Insights On Unsafe Peptide Practices

- Using peptides that have strong side effects

- Improper injecting techniques without a doctor's prescription

- Lack of breaks in between.

How Are Peptides Made?

- Peptides are formed when two or more amino acids create a bond, known as a peptide bond.

- Peptides can be synthesized in research or compounding pharmacy laboratories.

- Purchasing peptides from research labs tends to be more cost-effective. However, there may be some questions about their consistency and reliability.

- On the other hand, compounding pharmacy labs generally offer products at a higher price point but with a reputation for greater reliability.

- In some cases, peptides can be modified by adding a DAC (drug affinity complex), an amide group, or polyethylene glycol, among others. These modifications aim to prolong the peptide's presence in the bloodstream and enhance its efficacy.

- It is essential to understand how each peptide is made to get a comprehensive view of its benefits and side effects.

The Different Types of Peptides

- Pill

  - ¤ Most commonly, BPC-157, KPV, TB-4. I usually avoid pill peptides since most of the peptides will get destroyed in your stomach acid.

- Intra-Nasal

  - ¤ They are most commonly used for peptides that target your brain and cognitive function since they can pass the blood-brain barrier.

- Injectable

  - ¤ This is the most common way to administer peptides since they can enter the bloodstream effectively. Most peptides are injected subcutaneously (under the skin), while some peptides require intra-muscular (in the muscle)

- Topical

  - ¤ Most common with cosmetic peptides, like GHK-Cu and PTD-DBM, to directly target an area.

When To Take Peptides?

- Around 30, our bodies tend to produce fewer signaling agents, including peptides.

- From another standpoint, peptides may not be worthwhile if your body is in equilibrium.

- Peptides can be a significant financial burden. Therefore, I've always supported prioritizing lifestyle modifications and biohacking endeavors before turning to peptides.

20

- That said, I recognized the great potential of peptides as a supplementary element in a healthy routine, especially for those who were to start with subtle changes. As they progressed in other health aspects, they became more comfortable with peptide use, making delving deeper into this field, in that situation, a viable option. However, for those interested in peptides, it's crucial not to neglect other health facets or overlook the diverse impacts of money on your well-being.

Where To Buy Peptides

- Research Grade

  - These come in powder form and will have to be reconstituted.

  - Sigma Compounds is the current research institute I use to source peptides

- Compounding Pharmacy

  - You must go through a physician. The peptides come constituted. The quality may be more reliable but much more expensive, and you will have less control over the cycle since you will be working with a physician.

When Will You Start Seeing Results

- On average, it took me around two weeks to start noticing changes

- The timeline varied depending on my and other people's health, lifestyle choices, sensitivity, and the specifics of my peptide protocol (though higher dosages and frequency might hasten results, quicker isn't always better for others).

- Patience is key, where substantial results manifest after 6-8 months. Peptides aren't a miracle cure; they enhance natural body functions.

Do You Need an Off-Cycle with Peptides?

- I find off-cycles crucial for various reasons, including avoiding receptor overuse and assessing my body's response without peptide influence. It's also a financially savvy strategy, offering a chance to recalibrate future cycles based on my evolving goals.

- Unlike exogenous substances like hormones, which might suppress the body's natural functions, peptides aim to bolster existing bodily processes.

How To Maximize Peptide Effects?

- Prioritizing optimal lifestyle choices proved pivotal.

- Timing the peptide intake to coincide with specific goals to enhance their efficacy:

  - Example: Growth hormone peptides before a workout are said to be beneficial for fat burning.

  - Example: Post-workout growth hormone peptides are said to be beneficial for building muscle.

  - Example: BPC-157, whether before bed or post-exercise, could aid in recovery.

- Adjusting the dosage and frequency might offer additional benefits for those interested in learning about peptide use; though more isn't always better, costs can escalate.

- My mantra was to use peptides judiciously, only when truly necessary.

2. Peptides For Fat Loss

5-Amino-1-MQ

Overview

- 5-Amino-1-MQ is an oral peptide that is most commonly used to help reduce fat

- It mostly targets white adipose tissue by inhibiting the NNMT enzyme, leading to higher levels of NAD+, which has a cascade of benefits, one being weight loss.

- High levels of NNMT enzyme have been linked to obesity, type 2 diabetes, and overall, several metabolic complications.

How Does It Work?

- As people acquire more fat, they overproduce the enzyme NNMT. This enzyme slows down the rate at which the body can burn fat. As these cycles continue, more hormones and pro-inflammatory signals occur for weight gain, leading to chronic diseases such as type 2 diabetes.

- 5-Amino-1-MQ blocks the activity of NNMT. This creates an increase in NAD+, which is crucial for a wide array of cellular processes, one being the metabolic rate

- Blocking NNMT allows cells to use available energy (fat) more rapidly, resulting in fat reduction. Blocking NNMT allows the body to be less prone to storing fat

- 5-Amino-1-MQ helps activate the SIRT1 gene, also known as the "longevity gene," which significantly prevents diseases and bodily dysfunctions.

Research Benefits

- Promotes weight loss, especially in fat cells

- Improves energy levels

- Lowers cholesterol levels

- Improves blood sugar levels

- Fights inflammation

- Combats various cancer types

- Enhances aged muscle regeneration

Research Side Effects

- Difficulty sleeping

- Difficulty participating in exercise

Matthew's Personal Insight Research Cycling & Dosing

- 50-150 mg, taken all at once or split up

- It is essential to take with food due to 5-Amino-1-MQ being oil-solubility

- It is ideal to take it in the morning to prevent sleep disturbances

- Best to do cycles between 3-6 weeks long, with 1-2 week breaks in between to maximize potency

Peptides & Supplements Matthew Would Stack With

- Any GHRP (GHRP-2, GHRP-6, Ipamorelin, Hexarelin)

- Any GHRH (CJC-1295, MOD-GRF-1295, Tesamorelin)

- AOD-9604

- Semaglutide/Tirezepatide

- PEG-MGF

- Kisspeptin-10

- IGF-LR3

- Natural Diuretic (reduces water retention)

- Masculine Medicine

Pros & Cons

Pros

- Oral peptide

- Increases NAD+, which plays a major role in many cellular processes

- It can help someone get out of a rut when it comes to weight loss

Cons

- It can be expensive if taken on a continued basis

Matthew's Opinion

- This is one peptide I plan to take soon, as the increase in NAD+ seems promising. I would cycle with this 2-3 times a year.

- This would be a great peptide to take on a cut to enhance fat-burning effects and preserve muscle mass.

- The major downside is the cost. If cost is not an issue, this peptide is excellent to add to a stack whether to lose weight, prevent muscle breakdown, and/or experience several anti-aging benefits.

AOD-9604/Frag-176-191

Overview

- Anti-Obesity Drug-9604 (AOD-9604) is a synthetic growth hormone amino acid fragment.

- It contains similar but more potent fat-burning effects than growth hormone.

- Frag-176-191 is less stable and less effective than AOD-9604. Many peptide companies will market these in the same way.

How Does It Work?

- AOD 9604 works by enhancing lipolysis (breakdown of fat) and inhibiting lipogenesis (preventing fat storage)

- AOD-9604 fat-burning effects are unique as it does not enhance hunger, blood sugar levels, or tissue growth, which many growth hormone treatments can

- Additionally, AOD-9604 does not use the hGH receptor on the pituitary gland, as it acts independently of that. This makes it a potent peptide to stack with other GH peptides.

Research Benefits

- Helps regulate fat metabolism by stimulating lipolysis' (breakdown of fat) and inhibiting lipogenesis (transformation of food into body fat)

- It has other regenerative properties since it comes from the growth hormone amino acid.

- It doesn't compete with growth hormone receptors (essential for adding in other peptides)

- Reduces body fat

- Triggers fat release from obese fat cells predominantly more than lean ones

- Mimics the way natural growth hormone regulates fat metabolism

- No adverse effects on blood sugar or growth

Research Side Effects

- Redness, itchiness, and swelling of injection sites

Matthew's Personal Insight Research Cycling & Dosing

- 250-300 mcg, 1-2x daily through a subcutaneous injection

- It can be taken for 6 weeks or up to 6 months at a continuous dose

- It is best to take this peptide on an empty stomach in the morning or before a workout to maximize the fat-burning effects

- Some theorize injecting to the area where you want to reduce fat for more local benefits.

Peptides & Supplements Matthew Would Stack With

- Any GHRP (GHRP-2, GHRP-6, Ipamorelin, Hexarelin)

- Any GHRH (Tesamorelin, CJC-1295, MOD-GRF-129)

- BPC-157

- Semaglutide/Tirezepatide

- IGF-LR3

- MOTS-C

- Kisspeptin-10

- 5-Amino-1-MQ

- Masculine Medicine

Pros & Cons

Pros

- Targets fat metabolism specifically

- It can stack with other GH peptides and fat-burning peptides

- High safety profile

Cons

- Limited clinical results

Matthew's Opinion

- It is hard to say how effective this peptide is. I have stacked it with Ipamorelin and MOD-GRF-1295 multiple times.

- I did notice I sweat more when I do take it, meaning something is working

- Since this peptide is not too expensive and has a high safety profile, it makes a noteworthy peptide to add to a fat-burning stack

CJC-1295

- CJC-1295 is a GHRH (Growth Hormone Releasing Hormone)

- Contain DAC (drug affinity complex)

- Stays in the body for 6-8 days

- Enhances endogenous growth hormone in the body

How Does It Work?

- CJC-1295 goes up to the anterior pituitary gland and signals the body to create growth hormone (does not mean it will be released at the same time)

- Somatostatin is the rate-limiting effect that allows the release of growth hormone.

- By inhibiting somatostatin, the body is able to to release growth hormone (GHRP's does this)

- It is important to combine a GHRH with a GHRP to ensure the creation and release of growth hormone co-occurs.

- Less concerned about GHRP since CJC-1295 stays in the body for multiple days.

Research Benefits

- Increase production of endogenous growth hormone

- Promotes muscle growth

- Helps with mood and stress resilience

- Slows down aging

- Improves sleep

- Promotes a balanced inflammatory response

- Improves bone density

Research Side Effects

- Redness, itchiness, and swelling of injection sites

- Water retention

Matthew's Personal Insight Research Cycling & Dosing

- 100 mcg per injection (more is not better)

- Twice a week

- Daily injections can lead to HG levels above normal physiological levels

- 6-8 weeks on, 4-8 weeks off

- Carbohydrates and fatty acids can blunt growth hormone release. It is best taken 30 minutes before eating and/or 2 hours after eating

Matthew's Personal Insight on Timing & Benefits

- Timing matters less with this peptide since it stays in your body for 6-8 days.

- However, it is best to take each injection on an empty stomach

Peptides & Supplements Matthew Would Stack With

- Any GHRP (GHRP-2, GHRP-6, Ipamorelin, Hexarelin)

- BPC-157

- AOD-9604

- Semaglutide/Tirezepatide

- PEG-MGF

- Kisspeptin-10

- 5-Amino-1-MQ

- Natural Diuretic (reduces water retention)

- Masculine Medicine

Pros & Cons

Pros

- Requires few injections

- Increase GH with few side effects

Cons

- Unnatural how it stays on receptors for 6-8 days

Matthew's Opinion

- I use MOD-GRF-1-29 (CJC-1295 without DAC). I do not like having a peptide stimulate the receptors for multiple days.

- It is an all-around great peptide and is well used, especially when stacked with a GHRP (Ipamorelin is my favorite)

- This can be a great GHRH if the researcher wants a peptide with few injections or to increase GH levels quickly.

- I would stick with MOD-GRF-1-29 since it mimics our body's natural GH response.

MOD-GRF -1-29

Overview

- MOD-GRF-1-29 is a GHRH (Growth Hormone Releasing Hormone)

- It does not contain DAC (drug affinity complex)

- Half-life is around 30 minutes

- The most commonly used GHRH peptide

- Enhances endogenous growth hormone release in the body

How Does It Work?

- MOD-GRF-1-29 goes up to the anterior pituitary gland and signals the body to create more growth hormone (does not mean it will be released at the same time)

- Somatostatin is the rate-limiting effect that allows the release of growth hormone.

- By inhibiting somatostatin, the body is able to release growth hormone (GHRP's does this)

- It is important to combine a GHRH with a GHRP to ensure the creation and release of growth hormone co-occurs.

Research Benefits

- Increase production of endogenous growth hormone

- Promotes muscle growth

- Helps with mood and stress resilience

- Slows down aging

- Improves sleep

- Promotes a balanced inflammatory response

- Improves bone density

Research Side Effects

- Redness, itchiness, and swelling of injection sites

- Water retention

Matthew's Personal Insight Research Cycling & Dosing

- 100 mcg per injection (more is not better)

- Multiple injections can be given a day to increase GH secretion. Often used in bodybuilding

- 5 days on, 2 days off, 10-12 weeks on, 4-8 weeks off

- Carbohydrates and fatty acids can blunt growth hormone release. Best taken 30 minutes before eating and/or 2 hours after eating

Matthew's Personal Insight on Timing & Benefits

- Burning Fat

  ¤ Before a workout in a fasted state

- Building Muscle

  ¤ After a workout in a fasted state

- Sleep

  ¤ Before bed in a fasted state

- General Anti-Aging

  ¤ In the morning in a fasted state

Peptides & Supplements Matthew Would Stack With

- Any GHRP (GHRP-2, GHRP-6, Ipamorelin, Hexarelin)

- BPC-157

- AOD-9604

- Semaglutide/Tirezepatide

- PEG-MGF

- Kisspeptin-10

- 5-Amino-1-MQ

- Natural Diuretic (reduces water retention)

- Masculine Medicine

Pros & Cons

Pros

- The most commonly used GHRH with a high safety profile

- Follows how the pituitary naturally releases GH

Cons

- It is important to pair with a GHRP to get the most benefits

Matthew's Opinion

- This is one of my favorite GHRH

- I like how it mimics how the body naturally creates and releases GH

- It pairs well with Ipamorelin and is one of my favorite starter peptide blends

- It is all around great peptide and is well used, especially when stacked with a GHRP (Ipamorelin is my favorite)

Ipamorelin

Overview

- Ipamorelin is the mildest of GHRPs (Growth Hormone Releasing Peptide)

- Stimulates the release of growth hormone without an increase in appetite, cortisol, or prolactin

- Higher doses do not lead to desensitization

How Does It Work

- Ipamorelin works by inhibiting somatostatin in the hypothalamus

- Somatostatin is the rate-limiting effect that allows the release of growth hormone

- By inhibiting somatostatin, it allows the body to release growth hormone

Research Benefits

- Increase release of endogenous growth hormone

- Promotes muscle growth

- Helps with mood and stress resilience

- Slows down aging

- Improves sleep

- Promotes a balanced inflammatory response

- Improves bone density

Research Side Effects

- Redness, itchiness, and swelling of injection sites

- Water retention

- Facial flushing

Matthew's Personal Insight Research Cycling & Dosing

- 100 mcg per injection is the starting dose

- Multiple injections can be given a day to increase GH secretion. Often used in bodybuilding

- 5 days on, 2 days off, 10-12 weeks on, 4-8 weeks off

- Carbohydrates and fatty acids can blunt growth hormone release. Best taken 30 minutes before eating or 2 hours after eating

Matthew's Personal Insight on Research Timing & Benefits

- Burning Fat

  ¤ Before a workout in a fasted state

- Building Muscle

  ¤ After a workout in a fasted state

- Sleep

  ¤ Before bed in a fasted state

- General Anti-Aging

  ¤ In the morning in a fasted state

Peptides & Supplements Matthew Would Stack With

- Any GHRH (Tesamorelin, MOD-GRF, Sermorelin)

- BPC-157

- AOD-9604

- Semaglutide/Tirezepatide

- PEG-MGF

- Kisspeptin-10

- 5-Amino-1-MQ

- Natural Diuretic (reduces water retention)

- Masculine Medicine

Pros & Cons

Pros

- GHRP with a high safety profile

- Larger doses can be given without desensitization

Cons

- Mildest of the GHRPs

Matthew's Opinion

- My favorite GHRP

- I like how it increases GH without increasing other hormones

- A great GHRP for beginners since it has a high safety profile

Sermorelin

Overview

- Sermorelin is a GHRH (Growth Hormone Releasing Hormone)

- First FDA-approved GHRH used to address short status

- Enhances endogenous growth hormone release in the body

How Does It Work?

- Sermorelin goes up to the anterior pituitary gland and signals the body to create growth hormone (does not mean it will be released)

- Somatostatin is the rate-limiting effect that allows the release of growth hormone.

- By inhibiting somatostatin, it allows the body to release growth hormone (GHRP's does this)

- Combining a GHRH with a GHRP is important to ensure the creation and release of growth hormone co-occurs.

Research Benefits

- Increase production of endogenous growth hormone

- Promotes muscle growth

- Helps with mood and stress resilience

- Slows down aging

- Improves sleep

- Promotes a balanced inflammatory response

- Improves bone density

Research Side Effects

- Redness, itchiness, and swelling of injection sites

- Water retention

Matthew's Personal Insight on Research Cycling & Dosing

- 100-300 mcg per injection (1 mcg per kg)

- Multiple injections can be given a day to increase GH secretion. Often used in bodybuilding

- 5 days on, 2 days off, 10-12 weeks on, 4-8 weeks off

- Carbohydrates and fatty acids can blunt growth hormone release. Best taken 30 minutes before eating and/or 2 hours after eating

Matthew's Personal Insight on Timing & Benefits

- Burning Fat

  ¤ Before a workout in a fasted state

- Building Muscle

  ¤ After a workout in a fasted state

- Sleep

  ¤ Before bed in a fasted state

- General Anti-Aging

  ¤ In the morning in a fasted state

Peptides & Supplements Matthew Would Stack With

- Any GHRP (GHRP-2, GHRP-6, Ipamorelin, Hexarelin)

- BPC-157

- AOD-9604

- Semaglutide/Tirezepatide

- PEG-MGF

- Kisspeptin-10

- 5-Amino-1-MQ

- Natural Diuretic (reduces water retention)

- Masculine Medicine

Pros & Cons

Pros

- First FDA-approved GHRH

- High safety profile

Cons

- Weakest among the GHRH

- Shorter half-life than MOD-GRF-1-29

Matthew's Opinion

- Many researchers use Sermorelin since it was the "first" FDA GHRH

- There are several better GHRHs

- I use MOD-GRF-1-29 and then Tesamorelin if money is not a barrier.

Semaglutide

Overview

- Semaglutide is an FDA-approved medication for type-2 diabetes that possesses fat-burning properties.

- Semaglutide falls into the category of a glucagon-like-peptide-1 receptor agonist (GLP-1 RA)

- At higher doses, Semaglutide promotes fat loss and helps suppress appetite.

How Does It Work

- Semaglutide mimics the GLP-1 hormone released in the gut in response to eating.

- This targets the brain centers that regulate appetite and works on the stomach to slow down gastric emptying, which gives the feeling of being fuller for longer.

- Semaglutide promotes the body to produce more insulin, which helps move sugar from the blood into the other body tissues, overall leading to better blood sugar control and use.

Research Benefits

- Promotes fat loss

- Manages appetite

- Fights type 2 diabetes

- Prevents cognitive decline

- Lowers blood pressure

- Lowers the risk of cardiovascular disease

Research Side Effects

- Abdominal pain

- Constipation

- Loss of appetite

- Hypoglycemia

Matthew's Personal Insight on Research Cycling & Dosing

- 250 mcg, 1x a week for the first 4 weeks

- Increasing the dose 250 mcg every 4 weeks

- Do not exceed 2400 mcg per dose

- More is not always better

Peptides & Supplements Matthew Would Stack With

- CJC-1295, MOD-GRF, Tesamorelin

- Ipamorelin, GHRP-2

- AOD-9604

- MOTS-C

- 5-Amino-1-MQ

Pros & Cons

Pros

- An FDA-approved medication used for diabetes

- Well-used and well-researched

- 1x injection per week

Cons

- No major cons noted

Matthew's Opinion

- An all-around great peptide to manage weight and appetite

- This is becoming a popular peptide due to its benefits and safety profile

- Tirezepatide is better since it works on both GLP-1 and GIP receptors with fewer side effects

Tirezepatide

Overview

- Tirezepatide is a synthetic modification of the glucose-dependent insulinotropic peptide (GIP)

- Tirezepatide is considered the successor to Semaglutide when it comes to weight loss.

- Tirezepatide works on GIP and GLP-1 receptors, while Semaglutide only works on the GLP-1 receptors.

How Does It Work?

- Tirezepatide works both on GLP-1 and GIP receptors

- GIP receptors

  - Increases insulin secretion & sensitivity (reduces blood sugar levels)

  - Improves fat metabolism and triglyceride clearance

  - Prevents fat storage

- GLP-1 receptors

  - Enhances fat metabolism

  - Blunts appetite

  - Stimulates insulin released from the pancreas (lowers blood sugar levels)

Research Benefits

- Promotes fat loss

- Manages appetite

- Lowers blood sugar levels

- Fights type 2 diabetes

- Prevents cognitive decline

- Lowers blood pressure

- Reduces the risk of cardiovascular disease

Research Side Effects

- Abdominal pain

- Constipation

- Loss of appetite

- Hypoglycemia

Matthew's Personal Insight on Research Cycling & Dosing

- 2.5 mg, 1x a week for the first 4 weeks

- 5 mg, 1x a week for the second 4 weeks

- Best to cycle it 2-3x a year

Peptides & Supplements Matthew Would Stack With

- CJC-1295, MOD-GRF, Tesamorelin

- Ipamorelin, GHRP-2

- AOD-9604

- MOTS-C

- 5-Amino-1-MQ

Pros & Cons

Pros

- An FDA-approved medication used for diabetes

- Well-used and well-researched and more effective than Semaglutide

Cons

- Expensive

Matthew's Opinion

- An all-around great peptide to manage weight and appetite

- This is becoming a popular peptide due to its benefits and safety profile

- Tirezepatide would be my go-to weight-loss peptide

Tesamorelin

Overview

- Tesamorelin is a GHRH (Growth Hormone Releasing Hormone)

- FDA-approved drug for lipodystrophy (abnormal distribution of fat)

- The "Gold Standard" GHRH

- Enhances endogenous growth hormone creation in the body

How Does It Work?

- Tesamorelin goes up to the anterior pituitary gland and signals the body to create growth hormone (does not mean it will be released)

- Somatostatin is the rate-limiting effect that allows the release of growth hormone.

- By inhibiting somatostatin, it allows the body to release growth hormone (GHRPs do this)

- It is important to combine a GHRH with a GHRP to ensure the creation and release of growth hormone co-occurs.

Research Benefits

- Increase production of endogenous growth hormone

- Promotes muscle growth

- Helps with mood and stress resilience

- Slows down aging

- Improves sleep

- Promotes a balanced inflammatory response

- Improves bone density

Research Side-Effects

- Redness, itchiness, and swelling of injection sites

- Water retention

- Joint pain

- A sharp increase in IGF-1 levels

Matthew's Personal Insight on Research Dosing & Cycling

- 500-2000 mcg per injection

- Multiple injections can be given a day to increase GH secretion. Often used in bodybuilding

- 5 days on, 2 days off, 10-12 weeks on, 4-8 weeks off

- Carbohydrates and fatty acids can blunt growth hormone release. Best taken 30 minutes before eating or 2 hours after eating

Matthew's Personal Insight on Research Timing & Benefits

- Burning Fat

  ¤ Before a workout in a fasted state

- Building Muscle

  ¤ After a workout in a fasted state

- Sleep

  ¤ Before bed in a fasted state

- General Anti-Aging
  - ☐ In the morning in a fasted state

Peptides & Supplements Matthew Would Stack With

- Any GHRP (GHRP-2, GHRP-6, Ipamorelin, Hexarelin)

- BPC-157

- AOD-9604

- Semaglutide/Tirezepatide

- PEG-MGF

- Kisspeptin-10

- 5-Amino-1-MQ

- Natural Diuretic (reduces water retention)

- Masculine Medicine

Pros & Cons

Pros

- Strongest GHRH

- Maintains the negative feedback loop

- Strong benefits with a high safety profile

Cons

- Expensive

- Can sharply increase IGF-1 levels

Matthew's Opinion

- This is an excellent GHRH if money is not a limitation

- Combining this with Ipamorelin is considered the "Gold Standard" combo for increasing endogenous growth hormone

MOTS-C

Overview

- A gene in the mitochondrial DNA produces MOTS-C

- MOTS-C is often called the "exercise-induced" peptide

- This peptide plays a crucial role in signaling and energy production by regulating multiple metabolic functions throughout the body

How Does It Work?

- When MOTS-C is activated (either through stress or exercise), it moves to the nucleus and directs the nucleus's expression to promote cell balance.

- MOTS-C mainly acts on the AICAR pathway, which activates the AMPK pathway. AMPK plays a significant role in regulating growth, controlling autophagy (cell recycling), and metabolism

- The AMPK pathway has a robust downstream effect. It regulates energy metabolism, improves insulin sensitivity, reduces inflammatory responses, enhances fatty tissue activation, creates exercise-induced benefits, and protects the body against aging.

- Skeletal muscle is a primary target of MOTS-C due to its high concentration of mitochondria. When activated (as with normal exercise), the skeletal muscle enhances insulin sensitivity and increases muscle glucose uptake (without increasing insulin), leading to a healthier metabolism.

Research Benefits

- Accelerates weight loss

- Improves blood sugar levels and treats symptoms of diabetes

- Improves heart health

- Fights bone loss

- Increases life expectancy

- Improves exercise tolerance

- Fights bacterial infection

Research Side Effects

- Redness, itchiness, and swelling of injection sites

- Water retention

Matthew's Personal Insight on Research Dosing & Cycling Cycling

- 5mg three times a week (M/W/F) for 4-6 weeks

- Reduce down to 5mg once a week for 4 weeks

- Break for 4-6 weeks

Matthew's Personal Insight on Research Timing & Benefits

- Best to be taken in the morning or before a workout

Peptides & Supplements Matthew Would Stack With

- Any GHRP (GHRP-2, GHRP-6, Ipamorelin, Hexarelin)

- Any GHHR (Tesamorelin, CJC-1295, MOD-GRF-129)

- AOD-9604

- Semaglutide/Tirezepatide

- Humanin

- ARA-290

- SS-31

- Kisspeptin-10

- 5-Amino-1-MQ

- Masculine Medicine

Pros & Cons

Pros

- Naturally found in the body and has a multitude of benefits

- Most commonly used mitochondrial peptide

Cons

- Can be expensive

Matthew's Opinion

- This would be my go-to mitochondrial peptide. I like how it is found naturally in the body and has the most benefits compared to the other mitochondrial peptides.

3. Peptides For Building Muscle

DSIP

Overview

- DSIP stands for Delta Sleep-Inducing Peptide

- A similar peptide is found in large concentrations in human mother's milk

- Addresses sleep disturbances

- Resets circadian clock

- Supports the nervous system and hormonal system

How Does It Work?

- DSIP works by targeting several sites of the brain and brainstem that are linked to sleep and relaxation

- It interacts with the hormones serotonin, melatonin, and the neurotransmitter GABA, which all play a crucial role in falling and staying asleep.

- DSIP has been shown to increase endocrine functions during sleep, leading to higher releases of growth hormone, thyroid hormone, and testosterone

Research Benefits

- Improves sleep quality

- Reduces chronic pain

- Fights stress

- Boosts brain power

- Can help with depression

- Provides support for alcohol and opioid withdraw

- Stimulates LH (Luteinizing Hormone) and GHRH (Growth Hormone Releasing Hormone)

Research Side Effects

- Redness, itchiness, and swelling of injection sites

- Headache

- May disrupt sleep

- Dizziness

Matthew's Personal Insight on Research Dosing & Cycling

- 100 mcg 3 hours before bed daily

- Continue with dose based on response

- The goal is to restore normal sleep patterns

- Reduce down to 50 mcg 1x week once sleep stabilizes

Peptides & Supplements Matthew Would Stack With

- Any GHRP (GHRP-2, GHRP-6, Ipamorelin, Hexarelin)

- Any GHRH (CJC-1295, MOD-GRF-1, Tesamorelin)

- BPC-157

- TB-4

- TA-1

- PEG-MGF

- Kisspeptin-10

- Natural Diuretic (reduces water retention)

- Masculine Medicine

Pros & Cons

Pros

- Peptide designed for sleep

- It has additional benefits, such as helping increase growth hormone and testosterone

- High safety profile and relatively inexpensive

Cons

- It can disturb sleep if not dosed properly

Matthew's Opinion

- I have personally used this peptide and experienced longer and deeper sleep

- I also overdid and had the opposite effect

- Overall, I love this peptide, and it can be a great peptide to enhance the sleep

- More is not better with this peptide.

GHRP-2

Overview

- GHRP-2 is the second strongest GHRP (Growth Hormone Releasing Peptide)

- Stimulates the release of growth hormone & ghrelin (hunger hormone)

- Weakly and temporarily increases prolactin and cortisol

How Does It Work?

- GHRP-2 works by inhibiting somatostatin in the hypothalamus

- Somatostatin is the rate-limiting effect that allows the release of growth hormone

- By inhibiting somatostatin, it allows the body to release growth hormone

Research Benefits

- Increase the release of endogenous growth hormone.

- Promotes muscle growth

- Helps with mood and stress resilience

- Slows down aging

- Improves sleep

- Promotes a balanced inflammatory response

- Improves bone density

Research Side Effects

- Redness, itchiness, and swelling of injection sites

- Water retention

- Stimulates ghrelin, the hunger hormone (less than GHRP-6)

- Prolonged use and over-saturation of receptors may increase anxiety and depression.

- Increases in stress responses through an increase in prolactin, ACTH, and cortisol

Matthew's Personal Insight on Research Cycling & Dosing

- 100 mcg per injection

- Multiple injections can be given a day to increase GH secretion. Often used in bodybuilding

- 5 days on, 2 days off, 10-12 weeks on, 4-8 weeks off

- Carbohydrates and fatty acids can blunt growth hormone release. Best taken 30 minutes before eating and/or 2 hours after eating

Matthew's Personal Insight on Research Timing & Benefits

- Burning Fat
  - ¤ Before a workout in a fasted state

- Building Muscle
  - ¤ After a workout in a fasted state

- Sleep

  - ¤ Before bed in a fasted state

- General Anti-Aging

  - ¤ In the morning in a fasted state

Peptides & Supplements Matthew Would Stack With

- Any GHRH (Tesamorelin, MOD-GRF, Sermorelin)

- BPC-157

- AOD-9604

- Semaglutide/Tirezepatide

- PEG-MGF

- Kisspeptin-10

- 5-Amino-1-MQ

- Natural Diuretic (reduces water retention)

- Masculine Medicine

Matthew's Opinion

- This could be a good option if building mass is the main goal. It is safer and less aggressive than Hexarelin

- It also has less appetite stimulation than GHRP-6 with a more robust GH release

- Besides all of this, Ipamorelin is my go-to GHRP

GHRP-6

Overview

- GHRP-6 is the third strongest GHRP (Growth Hormone Releasing Peptide)

- Stimulates the release of growth hormone & ghrelin (hunger hormone)

- Weakly and temporarily increases prolactin and cortisol

How Does It Work?

- GHRP-6 works by inhibiting somatostatin in the hypothalamus

- Somatostatin is the rate-limiting effect that allows the release of growth hormone

- By inhibiting somatostatin, it allows the body to release growth hormone

Research Benefits

- Increase the release of endogenous growth hormone.

- Promotes muscle growth

- Helps with mood and stress resilience

- Slows down aging

- Improves sleep

- Increase hunger

- Improves bone density

Research Side Effects

- Redness, itchiness, and swelling of injection sites

- Water retention

- Strongly stimulates ghrelin

- Prolonged use and over-saturation of receptors may increase anxiety and depression.

- Increases in stress responses through an increase in prolactin, ACTH, and cortisol

Matthew's Personal Insight on Research Cycling & Dosing

- 100 mcg per injection

- Multiple injections can be given a day to increase GH secretion. Often used in bodybuilding

- 5 days on, 2 days off, 10-12 weeks on, 4-8 weeks off

- Carbohydrates and fatty acids can blunt growth hormone release. Best taken 30 minutes before eating and/or 2 hours after eating

Matthew's Personal Insight on Research Timing & Benefits

- Burning Fat
  - ¤ Before a workout in a fasted state

- Building Muscle
  - ¤ After a workout in a fasted state

- Sleep
  - ¤ Before bed in a fasted state
- General Anti-Aging
  - ¤ In the morning in a fasted state

Peptides & Supplements Matthew Would Stack With

- Any GHRH (Tesamorelin, MOD-GRF, Sermorelin)
- BPC-157
- IGF-LR3
- PEG-MGF
- Kisspeptin-10
- 5-Amino-1-MQ
- Natural Diuretic (reduces water retention)
- Masculine Medicine

Pros & Cons

Pros

- Strong GHRP with prolactin and cortisol increase less than GHRP-2 and Hexarelin
- Stimulates appetite

Cons

- Increase prolactin, cortisol, and appetite, ACTH (controls the production of cortisol)

Matthew's Opinion

- This could be a good option if building mass is the main goal. It is safer and less aggressive than Hexarelin and GHRP-2

- The increase in hunger could be seen as a benefit if the subject has trouble with consuming adequate calories for growth

Hexarelin

Overview

- Hexarelin is the most potent GHRP (Growth Hormone Releasing Peptide)

- Stimulates the release of growth hormone without an increase in appetite

- Increase in cortisol and prolactin

How Does It Work?

- Hexarelin works by inhibiting somatostatin in the hypothalamus

- Somatostatin is the rate-limiting effect that allows the release of growth hormone

- By inhibiting somatostatin, it allows the body to release growth hormone

Research Benefits

- Increase release of endogenous growth hormone

- Promotes muscle growth

- Helps with mood and stress resilience

- Slows down aging

- Improves sleep

- Promotes a balanced inflammatory response

- Improves bone density

Research Side Effects

- Redness, itchiness, and swelling of injection sites

- Water retention

- High risk of desensitization

- Prolonged use and over-saturation of receptors may increase anxiety and depression.

- Increases in stress responses through an increase in prolactin, ACTH, and cortisol

Matthew's Personal Insight on Research Cycling & Dosing

- 100 mcg per injection

- Multiple injections can be given a day to increase GH secretion. Often used in bodybuilding

- 5 days on, 2 days off, 4-8 weeks on, 4-8 weeks off

- Carbohydrates and fatty acids can blunt growth hormone release. Best taken 30 minutes before eating and/or 2 hours after eating

Matthew's Personal Insight on Research Timing & Benefits

- Burning Fat

  ¤ Before a workout in a fasted state

- Building Muscle

  ¤ After a workout in a fasted state

- Sleep

- ⌗ Before bed in a fasted state
- General Anti-Aging
    - ⌗ In the morning in a fasted state

Peptides & Supplements Matthew Would Stack With

- Any GHRH (Tesamorelin, MOD-GRF, Sermorelin)
- BPC-157
- AOD-9604
- Semaglutide/Tirezepatide
- PEG-MGF
- Kisspeptin-10
- 5-Amino-1-MQ
- Natural Diuretic (reduces water retention)
- Masculine Medicine

Pros & Cons

Pros

- Strongest GHRP
- Does not stimulate appetite as much as GHRP-2 and GHRP-6

Cons

- Increase prolactin, cortisol, and appetite, ACTH (controls the production of cortisol)
- High risk of desensitization

Matthew's Opinion

- The high risk of desensitization and increased cortisol and prolactin makes me cautious of this peptide.

- I would only micro-dose this peptide to maximize the benefits and reduce the side-effects.

- I mostly experiment with Ipamorelin, and it is my favorite GHRP

PEG-MGF

Overview

- PEG-MGF is a split variant of IGF-1 (insulin-like growth factor) IGF-1 -> MGF

- It can be found in muscles, bones, tendons, brain, and heart tissues

- The primary focus is to promote faster recovery from muscle damage

- Adding PEG (polyethylene glycol) increases the half-life of MGF to 48-72 hours

- MGF's normal half-life is 5-7 hours

How Does It Work?

- IGF-1 is spliced due to its response to broken-down muscle tissue. One of the spliced products is MGF

- PEG-MGF enhances muscle regeneration, activation and proliferation of satellite stem cells. This results in faster muscle growth and repair

Research Benefits

- Promotes muscle repair

- Speeds up bone repair

- Stimulates muscle growth

- Prevents heart disease

- Protects against stroke

- Promotes cognitive health

Research Side Effects

- Redness, itchiness, and swelling of injection sites

- Blood pressure drop

- Edema

Matthew's Personal Insight on Research Cycling & Dosing

- 100-600 mcg per injection

- It can be split into separate 100 mcg injections to target different muscles

- Suq-Q or IM muscle injections

- 2-3x week, 8-10 weeks on, 4-8 weeks off

Matthew's Personal Insight on Research Timing & Benefits

- Since PGF-MGF is a variant of IGF-1, it is essential not to use pre-workout, as IGF-1 and PGF-MGF fight for the same receptors.

- Rest days are the best way to get the most out of PEG-MGF since IGF-1 will be lower.

- Post-workout is the 2nd best option

Peptides & Supplements Matthew Would Stack With

- Any GHRP (GHRP-2, GHRP-6, Ipamorelin, Hexarelin)

- Any GHRH (CJC-1295, MOD-GRF-129, Tesamorelin, Ipamorelin)

- BPC-157

- AOD-9604

- Semaglutide/Tirezepatide

- IGF-LR3

- Kisspeptin-10

- 5-Amino-1-MQ

- Natural Diuretic (reduces water retention)

- Masculine Medicine

Pros & Cons

Pros

- Requires few injections

- Significant peptide for muscle recovery without increasing IGF-1 levels (can be helpful if subject is using other GH peptides)

Cons

- Limited amount of clinical research

Matthew's Opinion

- This peptide can be significant if the sole focus is muscle recovery and growth.

- I like how it can be used when IGF-1 levels are low

- I would use this 1-2x week on my off days in conjunction with GH peptides

IGF-1 LR3

Overview

- IGF-1 LR3 is a derivative of IGF-1 (released from the liver in response to growth hormone)

- IGF-1 LR3 has a greater half-life & bioavailability than IGF-1

- IGF-1 half-life -> 12 hours

- IGF-1 LR3 half-life -> 30 hours

- Most commonly used for building muscle and burning fat

How Does It Work?

- IGF-1 LR3 works by binding to IGF-1 receptors on muscle cells

- This enhances protein synthesis and inhibits protein breakdown

- IGF-LR3 stimulates satellite cells, which play a crucial role in muscle repair and function

- IGF-LR3 works on insulin receptors to enhance glucose uptake and overall lead to a more significant fat-burning effect

Research Benefits

- Increase in lean muscle mass

- Improvement of athletic performance

- Improvement of muscle recovery and reduced recovery time

- Reduction of body fat

- Increased metabolism

- Regulation of fat storage and prompts fat to be used for energy production

Research Side Effects

- Redness, itchiness, and swelling of injection sites

- Joint and muscle pain

- Edema

- Side-effects related to elevated IGF-1 levels

- Desensitization of receptors

Matthew's Personal Insight on Research Cycling & Dosing

- 20-60 mcg per injection

- 5 days on, 2 days off, 3-6 weeks on, 3-6 weeks off

- Best taken with food

Matthew's Personal Insight on Research Timing & Benefits

- Since IGF-1 LR3 is independent of the growth hormone being released, it does not need to be taken on an empty stomach like how other growth hormone peptides require

- Post-workout with food will give the greatest muscle-building effects.

Peptides & Supplements Matthew Would Stack With

- BPC-157

- AOD-9604

- Semaglutide/Tirezepatide

- PEG-MGF

- Kisspeptin-10

- 5-Amino-1-MQ

- Natural Diuretic (reduces water retention)

- Masculine Medicine

Pros & Cons

Pros

- Strong way to replicate IGF-1 levels

- A way to replicate the benefits of HGH replacement therapy

Cons

- Side effects if not dosed properly

- Desensitization can happen

- Limited research and clinical use

Matthew's Opinion

- This is a potent peptide that I would only explore once the subject has more experience with peptides.

- I would use this peptide 2-3x a week, focusing on the lower dose and cycle schemes

MK0677

Overview

- MK-677 (Ibutamoren) belongs to the GHRP category and is a SARM (selective androgen receptor modulator)

- Effective oral form of GH and IGF-1 replacement therapy. Can lead to supra-physiological IGF-1 response

- One of the most popular compounds due to its oral administration

- Proper sourcing of this compound is essential due to oral administration

How Does It Work?

- MK-677 mimics the actions of ghrelin (hunger hormone) by binding to one of the brain's growth hormone secretagogue receptors

- This allows for the release of growth hormone.

- Desensitization and damage of receptors are possible with high doses and prolonged cycles

Research Benefits

- Increase in lean muscle mass

- Promotes fat loss

- Maintains a healthy skeletal frame

- Improves sleep quality

- Improves cognitive function

- Accelerates wound healing and tissue regeneration

- Maintains a healthy heart

- Improves sex drive and sexual function

Research Side Effects

- Redness, itchiness, and swelling of injection sites

- Joint and muscle pain

- Edema

- No longer use than 8-12 weeks to avoid internalization of the receptor

- Irreversible neurological damage

- A sharp increase in cortisol

Matthew's Personal Insight on Research Cycling & Dosing

- 12.5-25 mg on an empty stomach

- 25 mg is the typical dose. It can be split up into 2 doses

- 12.5 mg is recommended for females

- Month 1 - 5 days a week

- Month 2 & 3 - 3 days a week

- Carbohydrates and fatty acids can blunt growth hormone release. Best taken 30 minutes before eating or 2 hours after eating

Matthew's Personal Insight on Research Timing & Benefits

- Burning Fat

  ¤ Before a workout in a fasted state

78

- Building Muscle

    - ⌶ After a workout in a fasted state

- Sleep

    - ⌶ Before bed in a fasted state

- General Anti-Aging

    - ⌶ In the morning in a fasted state

Peptides & Supplements Matthew Would Stack With

- Any GHRH (Tesamorelin, MOD-GRF, Sermorelin, CJC-1295)

- BPC-157

- AOD-9604

- Semaglutide/Tirezepatide

- PEG-MGF

- Kisspeptin-10

- 5-Amino-1-MQ

- Natural Diuretic (reduces water retention)

- Masculine Medicine

Pros & Cons

Pros

- Strong way to increase IGF-1 levels

- Oral administration

Cons

- A lot of vendors sell fake compounds

- Desensitization and permanent neurological damage can happen

Matthew's Opinion

- This is a powerful compound that I have seen many overuse and run into serious side effects.

- I would use this compound at a 12.5 mg dose, 3-5x a week in 1-month cycles, and then take a 1-month break

- I would stick to Ipamorelin if the subject is unsure about MK-677 and wants a safer GHRP

4. Peptides For Longevity

Epithalon

Overview

- Epithalon is a synthetic peptide that reproduces the effects of epithalamion, a peptide found naturally in the pineal gland

- The primary function of this peptide is to increase the length and activation of telomeres.

- Enhanced length and activation of telomeres are linked to a longer and healthier lifespan

- Traditionally classified as a bio-regulator

How Does It Work?

- Epithalon primarily works in the pineal gland of the brain

- Epithalon increases the production of the enzyme telomerase, which helps cells reproduce telomeres

- Telomeres act as a cap protector of our DNA that becomes worn out through DNA replication

- Since Epithalon works on the pineal gland, there are many documented effects of restoration of melatonin levels and improvement in circadian rhythm health

Research Benefits

- Decelerates aging

- Increase telomerase activity and elongation

- Normalizes melatonin levels

- Improve insulin sensitivity

- Prevents and fight cancer

- Promotes quality sleep

Research Side Effects

- Redness, itchiness, and swelling of the injection site

- Difficulty sleeping

- Fatigue

- Headache

Matthew's Personal Insight on Research Cycling & Dosing

- 50-100 mg total

- 5-10 mg daily for 10-20 days

- Recommended 1-2x a year to optimize longevity

- It is essential to take this peptide through an injection. Any oral form will not be absorbed appropriately

Peptides & Supplements Matthew Would Stack With

- Thymalin

- Any GHRP (GHRP-2, GHRP-6, Ipamorelin, Hexarelin)

- Any GHRH (CJC-1295, MOD-GRF, Tesamorelin)

- TB-4

- TA-1

- BPC-157

Pros & Cons

Pros

- A peptide specifically designed to enhance longevity

- Multiple studies have shown positive longevity effects

Cons

- It is hard to say how effective peptide is when using

- It can be expensive to run

Matthew's Opinion

- This peptide all around seems promising

- I like how it works on the pineal gland, which can have a multitude of benefits, especially if the goal is focused on consciousness and spirituality

- This peptide takes longer to feel the "effects." It may be best to experiment with faster-acting peptides first

TB-4/TB-500

Overview

- Thymosin Beta-4 (TB-4) is related to thymosin, a hormone secreted by your thymus, with its primary function to produce T cells, which is an essential aspect of the immune system.

- TB-4 plays an essential role in the protection, regeneration, and remodeling of injured tissues by influencing the movement of tissues

- TB-500 is often referred to as "TB-4," but TB-500 is a synthetic fragment of one of the four binding domains of TB-4. TB-500's primary purpose is to promote healing of joints and muscles

How Does It Work?

- Thymosin Beta-4 works by binding to actin, which is a protein that influences the action and formation of most cells in our body. Enhancing the mechanism of actin, leads to faster healing time, especially in injured areas

- Additionally, binding to actin increases the number of immune system cells and decreases inflammatory substances (cytokine)

- There are 4 specific binding domains of TB-4. Specific fragments of TB-4 can be used for a more potent healing effect

    - 17-23: targets musculoskeletal repair (healing of joints, muscle, ligaments)

    - 1-15: reduces apoptosis, addresses cytotoxicity (cell death)

    - 1-4: anti-inflammatory, anti-fibrotic

    - 40-43: heart support/health

Research Benefits

- Boosts the immune system

- Improves heart health

- Improves liver health

- Accelerates wound healing

- Improves eye health

- Promotes nerve regeneration

- Improves brain health

- Improves lung health

- Improves blood pressure

- Promotes hair growth

Research Side Effects

- Redness, itchiness, and swelling of injection sites

- Temporary tiredness

Matthew's Personal Insight on Research Cycling & Dosing

- 300 mcg to 1-gram subcutaneous injection

- This can be taken daily for up to 3 months or until the condition resolves

- Cycle length depends on the health status and response to treatment

- Take a 1-month break if cycling is needed for long-term

Peptides & Supplements Matthew Would Stack With

- Any GHRP (GHRP-2, GHRP-6, Ipamorelin, Hexarelin)

- Any GHRH (CJC-1295, MOD-GRF-1295, Tesamorelin)

- BPC-157

- LL-37

- TA-1

- KPV

- ARA-290

- GHK-Cu

Pros & Cons

Pros

- Heavily used and well-researched peptide

- It affects several aspects of the body, giving it a wide ray of use

Cons

- Many peptide companies will not specify which TB-4 fragment they are offering

Matthew's Opinion

- TB-4 is a potent peptide that I have used and benefited from. I love how it affects the body in numerous ways

- I like how I can find a specific fragment to focus on a specific area of healing with this peptide

- All around, one of my favorite peptides for healing and recovery

BPC-157

Overview

- BPC-157 stands for body-protective compound. It was discovered in the human gastric juice

- Often called the "wolverine" peptide

- It is one of the most well-used and well-researched peptides, as it offers a wide range of healing benefits

- BPC-157 is neuroprotective (brain), cardioprotective (heart), gastroprotective (stomach), and musculoskeletal protective (joints, ligaments, and muscles)

How Does It Work?

- BPC-157 works by activating regeneration properties of the body and also preventing growth-inhibiting effects in several aspects of the body (brain, stomach, heart, joints, muscles, ligaments)

- BPC 157 enhances angiogenesis (formation of new blood vessels), which plays a crucial role in promoting healing and helping cells regenerate faster

- BPC-157 works on the brain-gut axis, which allows it to protect organs, heal ulcers, modulate neurotransmitter levels in the brain, and overall enhance cognitive functions

Research Benefits

- Accelerates wound healing

- Accelerates healing of soft tissue injuries

- Improves bone and joint health

- Improves digestive health

- Improves cognitive health

- Exerts anti-cancer properties

- Helps regulate blood pressure

- Increases growth hormone receptors

Research Side Effects

- Redness, itchiness, and swelling of injection sites

- Water retention

Matthew's Personal Insight on Research Cycling & Dosing

- General use: 400-600 mcg

- Oral use: 500-1000 mcg

- Injury: Split the dose into 200-300 mcg and inject around the area

- Cycle length depends on the health status and response to treatment

Matthew's Personal Insight on Research Timing & Benefits

- For Brain Health

  - Intranasal spray taken on an empty stomach

- For Stomach Health

  - Taking orally on an empty stomach

- For Joint/Muscle/Ligament Injury

⌑   Inject around the area, splitting the dose into 2 injections a day

Peptides & Supplements Matthew Would Stack With

- Any GHRP (GHRP-2, GHRP-6, Ipamorelin, Hexarelin)

- Any GHRH (CJC-1295, MOD-GRF-129, Tesamorelin)

- TB-4

- KPV/VIP/LL-37

- IGF-LR3

- Kisspeptin-10

- 5-Amino-1-MQ

- Semax/Selank/Cerebrolysin

- Natural Diuretic (reduces water retention)

- Masculine Medicine

Pros & Cons

Pros

- One of the most well-used and well-research peptides

- It affects several aspects of the body, giving it a wide way of use

- It can be taken in several forms (orally, intranasal, injection)

Cons

- No major cons noted

Matthew's Opinion

- BPC-157 is one of my favorite peptides that I have extensive experience with

- It stacks well with many peptides and is great to use by itself

- This is one of my go-to peptides, as almost any subject could benefit from BPC-157

Humanin

Overview

- Humanin is a peptide found naturally in the mitochondria and many other parts of the human body, such as the heart, kidney, brain, and skeletal muscles.

- This peptide was initially classified as a mitochondrial peptide, but it was later classified as a neuropeptide since it was shown to help with Alzheimer's disease

- This peptide has been linked to largely influencing the health span and lifespan. Humanin levels are seen to be higher in children than adults, especially low in adults who suffer from Alzheimer's and mitochondrial dysfunctions

How Does It Work?

- Humanin regulates mitochondrial status by acting against apoptosis (cell death). It does this by inhibiting the function of a protein called Bax.

- Bax is a protein that resides inactive in the cytosol (fluid of cells) but will participate in cell death during normal development and various diseases. When Bax protein is triggered, it will target the mitochondria, releasing harmful compounds. Humanin prevents the Bat targeting, resulting in mitochondrial protection.

- Humanin binds to receptors throughout the body, resulting in enhanced intracellular signaling. This enhances protection against harmful agents.

- Overall, Humanin plays a role in returning the body to optimal function during a metabolic stress response.

Research Benefits

- Boosts mitochondria functions

- Improves lifespan and health span

- Reduces the risk of cardiovascular and metabolic diseases

- Reduces inflammatory markers

- Protects neurons

- Protects healthy cells from cell death

Research Side Effects

- Redness, itchiness, and swelling of injection sites

- No major side effects reported

Matthew's Personal Insight on Research Cycling & Dosing

- Dosing varies greatly on this compound since there is limited clinical data

- The study done on this showed .04 mg/kg as the therapeutic dose

- Weigh 80kg -> 3.2 mg

- Weigh 90 kg -> 3.6 mg

- Weigh 100 kg -> 4 mg

- Frequency varies from every day to once a week through a subcutaneous injection

Peptides & Supplements Matthew Would Stack With

- MOTS-C
- BPC-157
- TB-4
- TA-1
- SS-31
- KPV
- LL-37

Pros & Cons

Pros

- Found naturally in humans and linked to increased health span and life span

Cons

- Limited clinical use and data on this peptide

Matthew's Opinion

- The peptide community is still understanding this peptide
- I like how it is found naturally in the body
- I would start with MOTS-C or this peptide if choosing a mitochondrial peptide.
- If choosing this peptide, I would always start on a lower frequency and intensity until the subject gets a better idea of how this peptide interacts with the body.

5. Peptides For Brain Function

Semax/N-Acetyl Semax

Overview

- Semax comes from the adrenocorticotropic hormone (ACTH), which is typically produced as a stress hormone

- This peptide induces the "good" parts of stress, leading to enhanced mental performance and a variety of other benefits

- N-Acetyl Semax (added amide group) is better absorbed, more potent, and has a longer half-life than Semax

How Does It Work?

- Semax triggers the release of brain-derived neurotrophic factor (BDFN)

- BDNF plays a vital role in the development of new neurons and the creation of synapses, leading to enhanced neuroplasticity (the brain's ability to adapt and learn)

- Semax reduces the breakdown of enkephalins, which helps the brain reduce pain, inflammation, and cancerous development

- Semax falls into the category of a melanocortin. Melanocortin's can bind to melanocortin receptors, which are found in numerous parts of the body. This is why this peptide can enhance brain, gut, and immunity functions

Research Benefits

- Increases BDNF

- Increases dopamine and serotonin signaling

- Improves stress resilience

- Protects neurons

- Improves physical performance and adaptation to high-intensity exercise

- Improves memory, focus, attention span, and verbal fluency

- Improves blood flow to the brain

- May facilitate lucid dreaming

- Boosts confidence and wellbeing

Research Side Effects

- Excess and prolonged use can lead to desensitization.

- Low mood and motivation once the effects wear off, so subjects with pre-existing mental health conditions should be cautious

- Hair loss

Matthew's Personal Insight on Research Cycling & Dosing

- 100-300 mcg through a subcutaneous injection

- 750-1000 mcg through an intranasal spray (preferred method)

- 6 weeks on, 6 weeks off

Matthew's Personal Insight on Research Timing & Benefits

- Best taken in the morning in a fasted state

- Peptides are allowed to cross the blood-brain barrier easier in the absence of insulin (carbohydrates in the blood)

Peptides & Supplements Matthew Would Stack With

- Any GHRH (CJC-1295, MOD-GRF, Tesamorelin)

- Any GHRP (Ipamorelin, GHRP-2, GHRP-6, Hexarelin)

- Cerebrolysin

- Dihexa

- PE 22-88

- FGL (L)

- Oxytocin

- BPC-157

- TB-4

Pros & Cons

Pros

- A power neuropeptide with a wide range of benefits

- It can be easy to administer through an intranasal spray

Cons

- Causes hair loss

- It may give a "low" feeling after use

Matthew's Opinion

- This peptide is a powerful neuropeptide that helps with learning, mood, and overall health

- I do not like how it causes hair loss and can give a "low" feeling

- I would start with Selank or Cerebrolysin, especially if the subject was concerned about hair loss

Selank/N-Acetyl Selank

Overview

- Selank was created from Tuftsin (a peptide that naturally comes from the antibody immunoglobulin G) with additional sequins to enhance the peptides' stability.

- This peptide is often called the "anti-anxiety" peptide as it helps with learning, memory, depression, and energy.

- N-Acetyl Selank (added amide group) is better absorbed, more potent, and has a longer half-life than Selank.

How Does It Work?

- Selank works by regulating neurotransmitter levels in the brain, including serotonin, dopamine, and GABA. These all play a role in mood regulation and cognitive functions.

- Selank enhances BDNF, which plays a vital role in the development of new neurons and the creation of synapses, leading to enhanced neuroplasticity (the brain's ability to adapt and learn)

- Selank reduces the breakdown of enkephalins, which helps the brain reduce pain, inflammation, and cancerous development.

Research Benefits

- Increases BDNF

- Increases dopamine and serotonin signaling

- It can be used to help treat generalized anxiety disorder

- Enhanced learning and memory capacity

- Promotes healthy relaxation by increasing GABA

- Help with insulin resistance and metabolism

- It helps balance sleep vs wakefulness

- It helps regulate inflammation and has anti-viral properties

Research Side Effects

- Excess and prolonged use can lead to desensitization.

Matthew's Personal Insight on Research Cycling & Dosing

- 100-300 mcg through a subcutaneous injection

- 750-1000 mcg through an intranasal spray (preferred method)

- 6 weeks on, 6 weeks off

Matthew's Personal Insight on Research Timing & Benefits

- Best taken in the morning in a fasted state

- Peptides are allowed to cross the blood-brain barrier easier in the absence of insulin (carbohydrates in the blood)

Peptides & Supplements Matthew Would Stack With

- Any GHRH (CJC-1295, MOD-GRF, Tesamorelin)

- Any GHRP (Ipamorelin, GHRP-2, GHRP-6, Hexarelin)

- Cerebrolysin

- Dihexa

- PE 22-88

- FGL (L)

- Oxytocin

- BPC-157

- TB-4

Pros & Cons

Pros

- A power neuropeptide with a wide range of benefits

- It can be easy to administer through an intranasal spray

Cons

- No major cons noted

Matthew's Opinion

- This peptide is a powerful neuropeptide that helps with learning, mood, and overall health

- I like how it plays a role in regulating mood

- Selank or Cerebrolysin are my top peptides for cognitive enhancement

Cerebrolysin

Overview

- Cerebrolysin is a neuropeptide that comes from young pig brains

- It consists of many neuroactive vitamins, amino acids, and building blocks that support neuronal growth and function in and outside the brain.

- Cerebrolysin has a low molecular weight, allowing it to cross the blood-brain barrier readily

- Cerebrolysin has been around since the 1950s. It is an approved medication in 44 countries (not yet in the US)

How Does It Work?

- Cerebrolysin works by increasing the levels of neurotrophic factors (NFT), which restores damaged neurons and protects neurons from future damage

- Cerebrolysin protects neurons from free radicals, oxidative stress, acidosis, and neurotoxins by decreasing excitotoxicity (causes the death of central neurons), inhibiting free radical formation, and reducing neuroinflammation

- Cerebrolysin contains:

  - Nerve growth factors (promotes nerve regeneration)

  - BDFN (enhances growth of neurons)

  - P-21 (enhances DNA repair process)

  - Enkephalins (reduces pain, inflammation, and cancerous growth)

  - Orexin (improves learning, memory, and circadian rhythm health)

Research Benefits

- Improves energy production

- Helps treat concussions and TBIs

- Use to help Alzheimer's dementia

- Use to help with mood dysregulation

- Protects neurons from oxidative stress, excess acidity, and excess glutamate

- Reduces amyloid deposition

- Improves synaptic function

- Improves glucose uptake into the brain

- Helps with cognitive function and behavioral performance

Research Side Effects

- Dizziness

- Headache

- Sweating

- Nausea

Matthew's Personal Insight on Research Cycling & Dosing

- 5-10 ml (215 mg/ml) through a subcutaneous injection

- 10–20-day cycles

- Dosing intensity and frequency will vary with the subjects health status

Peptides & Supplements Matthew Would Stack With

- Any GHRP (GHRP-2, GHRP-6, Ipamorelin, Hexarelin)

- Any GHRH (CJC-1295, MOD-GRF-129, Tesamorelin)

- BPC-157

- TB-4

Pros & Cons

Pros

- Power neuropeptide that contains several neuroactive components

- Approved medication in 44 countries (not yet in the US)

Cons

- Can be expensive

Matthew's Opinion

- This is my favorite neuropeptide as it contains several powerful neuroactive compounds with a high safety profile

- If money were not a barrier, I would start with this peptide to enhance my cognitive health

PE-22-88

Overview

- PE-22-28 is a peptide derived from Spadin (a natural antidepressant peptide found in human blood)

- PE-22-28 blocks the TREK-1 channel in the brain. High levels of TREK-1 are associated with cognitive impairment and low mood.

- This peptide is being researched for use as a natural antidepressant, enhanced learning, stroke recovery, and neurodegenerative disease treatment.

How Does It Work?

- PE-22-28 binds to TREK-1 receptors in the brain. Blocking the TREK-1 channel

- TREK-1 is found in regions of the brain regulating mood, memory, and learning

- By reducing the levels of TREK-1, the body has a heightened ability to manage stress, memory recall, learning capabilities, and overall mood regulation.

- PE-22-28 is faster-acting and has a higher affinity (better binding) than most antidepressants. This allows for potent antidepressant benefits with a much higher safety profile than traditional antidepressants.

Research Benefits

- Improves mood and motivation

- Induces neurogenesis

- Improves firing rates of serotonin neurons

- Protects neurons from excess glutamate

- Improves the brain's stress resilience

- Preserves cognitive performance during stressful periods

Research Side Effects

- PE-22-28 is well-tolerated, and so far, no side effects have been reported

Matthew's Personal Insight on Research Cycling & Dosing

- 400 mcg intranasally

- 1x a day in the morning

Peptides & Supplements Matthew Would Stack With

- Any GHRP (GHRP-2, GHRP-6, Ipamorelin, Hexarelin)

- Any GHRH (CJC-1295, MOD-GRF-1295, Tesamorelin)

- BPC-157

- TB-4

- Semax/Selank/Cerebrolysin

- Selank

- Oxytocin

- FGL(L)

- Masculine Medicine

Pros & Cons

Pros

- Natural anti-depressant peptide with fast-acting benefits and high affinity. Making it much safer than most antidepressants

- Administered intranasally

Cons

- Limited clinical use

- Potentially can stimulate typical antidepressant side effects but at a lower degree

Matthew's Opinion

- This peptide is unique in its action. They took the natural antidepressant peptide (Spadin) decreased its half-life, and enhanced its potency.

- Because of its modification and the ability to be taken intranasally, I would try this peptide before using pharmaceutical antidepressants

- I would not use this long-term as I do not like the idea of its "blocking" a channel in the body. Short-term use with cycles would be how I would use it

Dihexa

Overview

- Dihexa was originally derived from angiotensin IV (a hormone naturally produced in our body that helps with memory)

- Dihexa has been reported to be 7x more potent than brain-derived-neurotrophic factor (BDFN), which has a multitude of benefits for the brain and body

- Dihexa is a powerful neuropeptide that has been shown to prevent the development of Parkinson-like symptoms and restore motor function.

How Does It Work?

- Dihexa binds to hepatocyte growth factor receptors (HGF), increasing HGF activity.

- HGF plays a significant role in preventing neuronal death and has several anti-inflammatory, pro-angiogenic (enhances blood cell formation), and immune-modulating benefits

- Dihexa can cross the blood-brain barrier, enhancing new synapses' formation.

- Dihexa has been said to be 7x more powerful than BDFN, which plays a major role in synapse formation.

- Dihexa has been shown to activate the PI3K/AKT pathway, which enhances synaptic plasticity and neuronal survival. These promote the restoration of nerve cells' structure and function, reduce inflammatory responses, and prevent nerve damage.

Research Benefits

- Helps with Alzheimer's disease

- Combats Parkinson's disease

- Improves learning and memory retention

- Improves stroke recovery

- Accelerates recovery from spinal cord injury and nerve damage

- Protects against hearing loss

Research Side Effects

- Jitters

- Irritability

- Mood swings

- Insomnia

- Long-term side effects uncertain

- Limited clinical data

Matthew's Personal Insight on Research Cycling & Dosing

- 10-50 mg taken daily either through powder or as a cream (rub onto inner forearms)

- Use no longer than 6 weeks

Peptides & Supplements Matthew Would Stack With

- Any GHRP (GHRP-2, GHRP-6, Ipamorelin, Hexarelin)

- Any GHRH (Tesamorelin, CJC-1295, MOD-GRF-1295)

- BPC-157

- TB-4

- Cerebrolysin

- Semax/Selank

- FGL(L)

- PE-22-88

Pros & Cons

Pros

- Powerful neuropeptide

- A similar variant is found naturally in the body

Cons

- Limited clinical use on the effectiveness and long-term safety

Matthew's Opinion

- It is a bit wild how Dihexa has been reported to be 7x more potent than brain-derived-neurotrophic factor (BDFN).

- I would start at the dosing scheme of Dihexa since it is a very powerful neuropeptide

- I also like how this peptide can be taken in powder or cream form

- I plan to experiment with this peptide myself soon

FGL (L)

Overview

- FGL(L) is a variant of the Neural Cell Adhesion Molecule (NCAM), which is found naturally on the surface of nerve cells (neurons) and glial cells (protect neurons)

- NCAM stimulates FGL, which helps produce new neurons and form new synapses between neurons

- This peptide contains several brain-protective and memory-enhancing properties.

How Does It Work?

- FGL directly increases fibroblast growth factor receptors, which increases neuronal growth and survival. This leads to enhanced memory.

- FGL increases AMPA receptor availability, which increases synaptic transmission, leading to faster information processing between neurons

- FGL activates the Protein Kinase C (PKC) pathway, which enhances synaptic plasticity. Synaptic plasticity is one of the key indicators of memory and learning capacity.

Research Benefits

- Improved cognitive function

- Helps heal traumatic brain injury

- Protection against neurotoxicity

- Improved memory

- Improved learning

- Prevents cognitive decline (Alzheimer's)

- Improvements in neuroinflammation

- Antidepressant features

Research Side Effects

- Redness, itchiness, and swelling of injection sites

- Limited clinical data

Matthew's Personal Insight on Research Cycling & Dosing

- 1-2 mg daily

- 5 days on, 2 days off

- Younger subjects in their 30's are recommended to do a lower dose (1mg or less)

Peptides & Supplements Matthew Would Stack With

- Any GHRP (GHRP-2, GHRP-6, Ipamorelin, Hexarelin)

- Any GHRH (Tesamorelin, CJC-1295, MOD-GRF-1295)

- BPC-157

- TB-4

- Cerebrolysin

- Semax/Selank

- Dihexa

- PE-22-88

Pros & Cons

Pros

- Powerful neuropeptide

- A similar variant is found naturally in the body

Cons

- Limited clinical use on the effectiveness and long-term safety

Matthew's Opinion

- This peptide interests me greatly. I like how it enhances neuron growth and synaptic formation.

- It gives the body more brain-building blocks and then helps connect them (that's how I think about it)

- It is hard to say how effective or safe this peptide is with the limited clinical use

- I plan to experiment with this peptide myself soon.

6. Peptides For Immunity

Thymosin-Alpha-1

Overview

- Thymosin Alpha 1 is a peptide that is naturally produced by the thymus gland

- This peptide plays a crucial role in the development of immune system cells (T-cells), which are vital in fighting bacteria, fungi, and viruses

- This peptide is given to patients with hepatitis B/C, HIV, cancer, Lyme, and a variety of autoimmune conditions.

How Does It Work?

- Thymosin alpha 1 stimulates signaling pathways in the immune system, producing and activating T-cells, dendritic cells, and natural killer cells.

- T-cells, dendritic cells, and natural killer cells play a vital role in fighting bacteria, fungi, and viruses

- Thymosin alpha 1 strengthens the immune system in numerous ways and addresses both aspects of the immune system (TH1-innate and TH2-acquired) immunity to help return to homeostasis.

Research Benefits

- Eradicates bacteria, viruses, and fungi

- Boosts the function of certain immune cells

- Suppresses cancer and tumor growth

- Accelerates the wound-healing process

- Fights inflammation

- Enhances antibody responses

- Balances TH1/TH2

Research Side Effects

- Redness, itchiness, and swelling of injection sites

- A very safe peptide

Matthew's Personal Insight on Research Cycling & Dosing

- 1-1.5 mg per subcutaneous injection

- Every third day

- 2 weeks to 3 months or longer. The cycle depends on the response and overall health status

Peptides & Supplements Matthew Would Stack With

- BPC-157

- TB-4

- ARA-290

- VIP

- KPV

- LL-37

Pros & Cons

Pros

- A powerful peptide to help strengthen the immune system

- Heavily researched and used with a high safety profile

- FDA approved

Cons

- It can be expensive if run long-term

Matthew's Opinion

- This is a powerful immune peptide that I would use as my first peptide to work on my immune health.

- It is low-risk with a high reward.

- Overall, it is one of the most effective and safest peptides, especially among the immunity peptides

LL-37

Overview

- LL-37 is antimicrobial, antiviral, and an anti-biofilm (fights off gram-positive and gram-negative pathogens)

- Humans produce this peptide naturally in their neutrophils, natural killer cells, and in many different body systems

- LL-37 has the potential to serve as an alternative to antibiotics and plays a vital role in innate and adaptive immunity

How Does It Work?

- LL-37 stimulates groups of responses in many cells, either directly or through the influence of cellular responses to microbial compounds

- LL-37 is released when neutrophils, natural killer cells, and macrophages are stimulated. These cells can be found in bone marrow, on the skin, on the gastrointestinal tract, and in your lungs

- LL-37 can interact with molecules on the cell wall, poking holes in the membranes resulting in bacterial cell death

- This results in a broad-spectrum defense against bacterial invasion

Research Benefits

- Prevents lung injury and fights lung infections

- Protects against gut inflammation from gut infections

- Helps call other immune cells to the site

- Promotes a balanced immune response

- Accelerates wound healing

- Promotes bone repair

Research Side Effects

- Redness, itchiness, and swelling of injection sites

- Increased inflammation

- Induction of autoimmune disease (high LL-37 is found in patients with autoimmune diseases)

- Damage to sperm surface membranes

- Toxic to both bacterial and normal cells

Matthew's Personal Insight on Research Dosing & Cycling

- 100 mcg per injection

- It can be given 2x a day. Once in the morning and once at night

- 4–6-week cycle and then evaluate patient's response and status

Matthew's Personal Insight on Research Timing & Benefits

- It is best taken when the body is fighting a serious infection

Peptides & Supplements Matthew Would Stack With

- BPC-157

- TB-4

- TA-1

- VIP

- KPV

Pros & Cons

Pros

- A powerful peptide to help strengthen the immune system

- Potential alternative to an antibiotic

Cons

- Can cause the opposite effects

- Limited clinical data

Matthew's Opinion

- This is a powerful immune peptide that I would only use if I were working closely with a doctor

- The risk of damaging my body and causing the opposite effect makes it risky

- I would not run this peptide long-term and only use it in the beginner phases of an infection

- I would start with other immune peptides (TB-4, TA-1), which are effective and much safer

KPV

Overview

- KPV is naturally produce in the body and is found in the hormone alpha-MSH

- KPV is most commonly used for autoimmune and inflammatory conditions

- This peptide can be used as a cream, injectable, or capsule. The route of administration depends on which area is being focused on

How Does It Work?

- KPV can enter cells and nuclei, where DNA is. Inside, it can inhibit NF-kB, one of the cell's main controllers of inflammation.

- KPV plays a role in inhibiting different microbes from forming

- Topical KPV has been shown to speed wound healing, reduce infection and inflammation

Research Benefits

- Inhibits NF-kB and inflammatory signaling

- Reduces inflammatory cytokines

- Promotes a balanced inflammatory response, especially in the gut

- Promotes wound healing

- It may have antimicrobial activities

- Improves skin health and regeneration

- Helps with Inflammatory Bowel Diseases (IBD) and colitis

Research Side Effects

- Redness, itchiness, and swelling of injection sites

- No side effects have been reported

Matthew's Personal Insight on Research Cycling & Dosing

- The goal is to use KPV until the condition is healed

- Subcutaneous: 200-500 mcg, one time a day

  ¤ Best used for overall inflammation

- Oral: 250 mcg, twice a day on an empty stomach

  ¤ Best used for any stomach/GI inflammation

- Topical: 7.5 mg applied 2x a day to area

  ¤ Best used for wound healing

Peptides & Supplements Matthew Would Stack With

- GHK-Cu

- BPC-157

- TB-4

- TA-1

- LL-37

- Humanin

Pros & Cons

Pros

- Can enter cells and shut down inflammatory pathways

- Multiple ways to be applied (injection, oral, topical)

Cons

- Limited clinical use and research

Matthew's Opinion

- This is one of the few peptides that can be applied in multiple ways

- Depending on it is administrated, it will give different benefits. This makes it a significant peptide to work on numerous health conditions

- This peptide is most commonly used for gut/GI conditions. I would use this peptide if I had any GI issues or any major topical wounds.

SS-31 (Elamipretide)

Overview

- SS-31 (Elamipretide) is a synthetic derived peptide that targets mitochondria and has been shown to protect and heal mitochondria

- Szeto-Schiller (SS) peptides target mitochondria membranes and are classified as a ROS (reactive oxygen specifics) scavenger, which prevents damage to cells

- SS-31 has several anti-aging effects that could help with the treatment of age-related diseases, genetic disorders, kidney injuries, and heart diseases

How Does It Work?

- SS-31 targets mitochondria, specifically the inner mitochondrial membrane, by binding to cardiolipin

- Cardiolipin is a phospholipid unique to the mitochondria that plays a major role in mitochondrial metabolism, protection, and function

- SS-31 binding to cardiolipin prevents oxidation (damage) of this protective mitochondrial phospholipid

- This leads to enhanced protection and restoration of the mitochondria, resulting in more ATP and improved cellular processes.

Research Benefits

- Improves cardiovascular health

- Boosts brain power

- Prevents cancer

- Prevents kidney injury

- Helps heal lung injuries

Research Side Effects

- Redness, itchiness, and swelling of injection sites

- Abdominal pain

- Dizziness

- Headache

Matthew's Personal Insight on Research Cycling & Dosing

- The dosage of SS-31 could be upwards of 40 mg per day through a subcutaneous injection

- The exact dosage depends on the reason for using the peptide

- The peptide does seem to be well-tolerated over a wide dose range

Peptides & Supplements Matthew Would Stack With

- Any GHRP (GHRP-2, GHRP-6, Ipamorelin, Hexarelin)

- Any GHRH (Tesamorelin, CJC-1295, MOD-GRF-129)

- BPC-157

- TB-4

- MOTS-C

- ARA-290

- 5-Amino-1-MQ

Pros & Cons

Pros

- Helps restore and protect mitochondria, leading to a cascade of benefits

Cons

- Peptide with limited clinical use

Matthew's Opinion

- This peptide seems like it could be beneficial in correcting mitochondrial dysfunction

- I would personally start with MOTS-C, a more well-known mitochondrial-enhancing peptide

- I would start at a lower dosing scheme and slowly increase in intensity and frequency depending on the response

ARA-290

Overview

- ARA-290 is a peptide designed off a segment of the hormone erythropoietin

- Its main mechanism of action focuses on tissue repair and protection

- Commonly used for patients with diabetes or suffering neuropathy (damage of nerves)

How Does It Work?

- ARA-290 comes from the hormone EPO (erythropoietin)

- It does not stimulate new red blood cells, which EPO does; instead, it stimulates tissue repair and protection through β-common receptors

- It promotes tissue repair and protection by activating the body's natural repair system by turning on the innate repair receptors and shutting down systemic inflammation

Research Benefits

- Promotes healthy blood sugar control

- Protects neurons from oxidative stress

- Protects heart tissues

- Promotes a balanced inflammatory response

- Relieves neuropathic pain

- Fights diabetes

Research Side Effects

- Redness, itchiness, and swelling of injection sites

- No side effects of ARA 290 have been reported in clinical trials

Matthew's Personal Insight on Research Cycling & Dosing

- 4mg/day through a subcutaneous injection

- 30-day cycles

- Based on the patient's response

Peptides & Supplements Matthew Would Stack With

- Any GHRP (GHRP-2, GHRP-6, Ipamorelin, Hexarelin)

- Any GHRH (CJC-1295, MOD-GRF, Tesamorelin)

- BPC-157

- TB-4

- TA-1

Pros & Cons

Pros

- Peptide specifically used for diabetic patients

- Shows promising results for patients who suffer from neuropathy

Cons

- It can be expensive to run

- Limited clinical use and research

Matthew's Opinion

- This peptide seems promising for diabetic patients

- A lot of treatments and medications for diabetic patients have serious side effects

- I would use this peptide if I wanted to explore alternative treatments for diabetes or if I was suffering from neuropathy

Vasoactive Intestinal Peptide (VIP)

Overview

- Vasoactive Intestinal Peptide (VIP) is a neuropeptide naturally found in the intestines, pancreas, brain, central nervous system, urogenital system, lungs, and all over the body

- It plays a significant role in blood circulation, energy production, and blood pressure regulation.

- Its main benefit is that it is a vasodilator, which enhances blood flow to all body parts, leading to improved function and health.

How Does It Work?

- VIP is prevalent across the body. This makes it difficult to know the exact mechanism of action.

- VIP acts as a vasodilator, allowing an increase in blood flow and smooth muscle relaxation. Blood is rich in oxygen and essential nutrients and has the benefits of cleaning waste. The new blood flow combined with smooth muscle relaxation can benefit every system in the body.

- VIP can help enhance blood flow to penile tissue, helping with erectile dysfunction (ED)

- VIP can enhance blood flow and relaxation to the lungs, helping COPD and asthma

- VIP works on the lymphatic and nervous system, allowing improved movement in lymph and enhanced immunity

Research Benefits

- Lowers the risk of heart disease

- Promotes healthy lungs

- Promotes wound healing

- Regulates blood pressure

- Promotes a healthy digestive system

- Prevents cancer

- Boosts immunity

- Helps with erectile dysfunction

Research Side Effects

- Dizziness

- Headaches

- Irritability

- Low blood pressure

- Rash

Matthew's Personal Insight on Research Cycling & Dosing

- 50 mcg sprayed in each nostril

- 1-16 times a day

- This peptide is fast-acting with a short half-life (2 minutes)

- It is best to use peptides when wanting to enhance blood flow or muscle relaxation

- Dosing frequency and intensity depends on the response and condition

- The goal is not to become dependent on the compound

Peptides & Supplements Matthew Would Stack With

- BPC-157

- TB-4

- ARA-290

- KPV

Pros & Cons

Pros

- It can be given through an intranasal spray

- Effects multiple parts of the body, giving it a wide way of use

Cons

- Does not work on the root cause of poor blood flow/performance

Matthew's Opinion

- I like how this peptide works on many aspects of the body

- I could see this being beneficial for supporting erectile dysfunction/ sexual performance or lung/breathing discomfort

- It is important to note that this peptide will not fix the root cause of the lack of performance/blood flow.

7. Peptides For Cosmetics

PTD-DBM

Overview

- PTD-DBM is a topical man-made peptide to fight hair loss

- PTD-DBM prevents hair loss and promotes the growth of new hair follicles by interfering with the CXXC5 protein binding

- This peptide is commonly paired with topical valproic acid since both work on the same pathway (Wnt/β-catenin pathway) to fight hair loss

How Does It Work?

- CCX5 is a protein that acts as a negative regulator of the Wnt/β-catenin pathway

- The Wnt/β-catenin pathway is linked to hair regeneration and wound healing

- PTD-DBM interferes with the binding of CCX5, allowing for hair regeneration and wound healing to happen

- Valproic acid is added to activate the Wnt/β-catenin pathway

Research Benefits

- Reduces Seizures

- Fights Hair Loss

- Helps With Migraines

- Improves Mood

- Improves Cognitive Function

- Accelerates Hair Regeneration

- Improves Wound Healing

Research Side Effects

- PTD-DBM is a relatively newer peptide, and more scientific literature is needed.

- Therefore, its side effects have yet to be explored.

Matthew's Personal Insight on Research Cycling & Dosing

- PTD-DBM sprays are usually available as a 0.001% solution in 25 ml of spray bottles

- Liquid forms of this peptide are also available in vials of 5 mg.

- Literature shows using topical spray 1-2x week

Matthew's Personal Insight on Research Timing & Benefits

- It is best to apply it after a shower. This will prevent the hair's natural oil from blocking the absorption of PTD-DBM.

- Absorption and hair growth can be enhanced by micro-needling before applying PTD-DBM.

- Valproic acid is recommended to apply with PTD-DBM for maximal benefits.

Peptides & Supplements Matthew Would Stack With

- Any GHRP (GHRP-2, GHRP-6, Ipamorelin, Hexarelin)

- Any GHRH (CJC-1295, MOD-GRF, Tesamorelin)

- TB-4

- BPC-157

Pros & Cons

Pros

- Powerful hair growth peptide that does not block DHT (rescue hair follicles instead)

- Safer, cheaper & more effective than most hair-loss solutions

- Promising results for those who've tried

Cons

- It does not address underlying inflammation or lack of blood flow to the scalp

- Limited clinical research

Matthew's Opinion

- This is one peptide I am pumped to experiment with

- The mechanism of action is unique in how it "saves" hair follicles

- I would make sure to combine this with scalp brushing, derma rolling, valproic acid, and red-light therapy to get the most out of this hair growth stack

GHK-Cu

Overview

- GHK-Cu is a naturally occurring copper peptide found in human plasma. As people age, they naturally lose the ability to produce this

- This peptide is commonly used in hair and skin products due to its strong regeneration and anti-inflammatory properties

- This peptide modulates over 500 different gene expressions, resulting in multiple health and anti-aging benefits

How Does It Work?

- GHK-Cu affects multiple pathways in the body, leading to a wide ray of benefits

- For tissue injuries, GHK-Cu acts as a chemoattractant (stimulating cell signaling and movement of cells during inflammatory actions) while releasing proteins to stimulate the growth and repair of tissue

- GHK-Cu increases collagen, stem cell production, and bone formation by stimulating chondrocytes in bones

- GHK-Cu provides a source of copper for cells, which copper is essential for angiogenesis (development of new blood cells), which plays a significant role in tissue growth and survival

- GHK-Cu blocks the release of oxidative damage released from ferritin channels after injury, allowing for enhanced regeneration properties for skin, hair follicles, stomach lining, bone tissue, fingernails, and many other aspects of the body

Research Benefits

- Tightens loose skin

- Enhances skin elasticity

- Reduces fine lines and wrinkles

- Accelerates wound healing

- Improves lung health

- Fights hair loss

- Accelerates nerve regeneration

- Promotes bone repair

- Fights Inflammation

Research Side Effects

- Redness, itchiness, and swelling of injection sites

- Possibility for copper toxicity

- Lunula of the nail can turn blue (corrects after 4-6 weeks)

- Do not mix with vitamin or Hyaluronic Acid when applying to skin for best results

Matthew's Personal Insight on Research Cycling & Dosing

- For subcutaneous injections: 1-2 mg per day

- For topical: any place to focus on healing

- 6-week intervals

- Can be cycled 3-4x a year

Matthew's Personal Insight on Research Timing & Benefits

- For hair and skin:
    - ¤ Best to apply after a shower. This will prevent the hair and skin's natural oil from stopping GHK-Cu from being absorbed
    - ¤ Absorption and results can be enhanced by micro-needling before applying GHK-Cu

Peptides & Supplements Matthew Would Stack With

- Any GHRP (GHRP-2, GHRP-6, Ipamorelin, Hexarelin)
- Any GHRH (CJC-1295, MOD-GRF-1295, Tesamorelin)
- BPC-157
- TB-4
- TA-1
- KPV
- ARA-290

Pros & Cons

Pros

- Regenerates several aspects of the body
- It can be used topically, orally, intranasally, and subcutaneously
- Heavily used and researched

Cons

- Topical compounds can be expensive

- It will take time to see significant results

Matthew's Opinion

- I have personally used GHK-Cu topically for hair growth, and my skin

- I saw some results but did not like how pricey the cosmetic GHK-Cu compounds were

- Overall, it is an excellent peptide to add to a cosmetic stack. I would start with GH peptides if the main goal was cosmetics and then add GHK-Cu once the budget increases

8. Peptides For Sexual Health

Kisspeptin-10

Overview

- Kisspeptin-10 is a neuropeptide hormone from the hypothalamus

- Often called the "puberty" peptide

- It helps normalize the sex hormone feedback loop

- Can enhance sexual arousal and fertility

How Does It Work?

- Kisspeptin-10 stimulates the release of GnRH (Gonadotropin Releasing Hormone) in the hypothalamus.

- This allows for the release of LH (Luteinizing Hormone) and FSH (Follicle Stimulating Hormone) in the pituitary.

- In men, LH and FSH signal the testes to create more testosterone and sperm

- In women, LH & FSH signals the ovaries to make more estrogen and signals the release of an egg (ovulation)

Research Benefits

- Increases sex hormones in both males and females (testosterone, estrogen)

- Enhances fertility

- Temporarily increases oxytocin

- Improves brain health and mental/emotional processing

- Prevents cancer

Research Side Effects

- Redness, itchiness, and swelling of injection sites

Matthew's Personal Insight on Research Cycling & Dosing

- 1 mcg per kg (100-200 mcg)

- Best taken in a fasted state in the morning to mimic natural testosterone production

- Peak FSH & LH occurs 45-60 minutes after injection

- 3-5x week, 1 month on, 1 month off

Matthew's Personal Insight on Research Timing & Benefits

- Testosterone Production (Men)

    - Best taken in the morning in a fasted state

- Fertility

- ¤ Women -> Best taken around regular ovulation and 45-60 minutes before attempting conception

- ¤ Men -> Best taken around 45-60 minutes before attempting conception

Peptides & Supplements Matthew Would Stack With

- Any GHRH (Tesamorelin, MOD-GRF, Sermorelin, CJC-1295)

- Any GHRP (Ipamorelin, GHRP-2, GHRP-6, Hexarelin)

- PT-141

- Melanotan-2

- IGF-LR3

- AOD-9604

- Semaglutide/Tirezepatide

- PEG-MGF

- 5-Amino-1-MQ

- Masculine Medicine

Pros & Cons

Pros

- Only peptide that works on the sex hormone axis

- Peptide specifically used to increase testosterone and fertility

- Pairs well with HRT therapy

Cons

- Limited research

Matthew's Opinion

- I have personally used this peptide on/off. It is hard to say how effective this peptide was without getting before/after blood work.

- The mechanism of action seems promising since it starts the testosterone cascade effect.

- Due to its low cost and high benefit profile, it would be worth looking into

Melanotan I & II

Overview

- Melanotan I and Melanotan II work on the melanocortin system and replicate the hormone melanocortin, which is naturally released by the pituitary gland

- These peptides increase melanogenesis, which plays an import role in tanning, immune support, and sexual support

- Melanotan I is often used more frequently as it has fewer side effects than Melanotan II

- Melanotan II does display a more intense response with more benefits but has a higher side-effect profile.

How Does It Work?

- Melanotan I mainly binds to the MC1R receptors.

- Melanotan II mostly binds to MC1R, MC3R and MC4R receptors

  - MC1R (melanogenesis -> tanning)

  - MC3R (suppression of appetite)

  - MC4R (enhanced sexual stimulus)

Research Benefits

- Helps with various skin disorders

- Supports immune system

- UV/tanning protection

- Increases libido and improves erectile function in men (Mostly Melanotan II)

- Cardio and neuroprotective

- Supports appetite and metabolism (Mostly Melanotan II)

- Helps with alcohol abuse disorder

Research Side Effects

- Sexual stimulation (erection lasting longer than 4 hours) - Mostly concerned with Melanotan II

- Can potentially increase blood pressure

- Nausea

- Vomiting

- Headache

- Do not use if there is a history of skin cancer

- Do not use with other PDE5 inhibitors (Viagra, Tadalafil) - Mostly concerned with Melanotan II

Matthew's Personal Insight on Research Cycling & Dosing

- For Tanning
  - 200 mcg daily for 1 week
  - 50-100 mcg 1-2x a week after reaching the skin-tone goal
- For Immunity
  - 200 mcg daily for 6-8 weeks
- For Metabolic Support
  - 50 mcg daily

- For Sexual Stimulation

  - ¤ 200-1000 mcg before intercourse

Peptides & Supplements Matthew Would Stack With

- Any GHRP (GHRP-2, GHRP-6, Ipamorelin, Hexarelin)

- Any GHRH (CJC-1295, MOD-GRF-1295, Tesamorelin)

- AOD-9604

- Semaglutide/Tirezepatide

- PT-141

- VIP

- Kisspeptin-10

- Masculine Medicine

Pros & Cons

Pros

- Melanotan I is FDA-approved

- Great peptides to increase skin tone

- Melanotan II can be beneficial for erectile dysfunction

Cons

- It takes more skill to use these peptides. Too much can lead to side effects

- It has more side effects than most peptides

Matthew's Opinion

- Melanotan I and Melanotan II are powerful peptides that, use in the right way, can be great

- I have personally used Melanotan II and like the tanning benefits, and I am still exploring the sexual benefits

- If I were new to peptides and wanted to focus on the tanning benefits, I would personally start with Melanotan I.

- Melanotan II can be harder to use since it is more intense with a higher side-effect profile

PT-141 (Bremelanotide)

Overview

- PT-141 is a libido-boosting peptide targeting the melanocortin receptors (MC3R and MC4R)

- Discovered from Melanotan-2

- Works on the nervous system rather than the cardiovascular system (most erectile drugs work on the cardiovascular system)

- This peptide can be taken through a subcutaneous injection or a nasal spray.

How Does It Work?

- PT-141 works on the MC4R and MC3R receptors in the hypothalamus

- This signals receptors in the central nervous system to enhance blood flow, libido, and arousal

Research Benefits

- Increases sexual desire, motivation, and arousal across genders

- Induces erectile response

- Improves genital sensation and pleasure

- It may help with discomfort and orgasm during intercourse

- It may help with emotional issues around sex

- Improves heart health and metabolism

- Promotes healthy blood pressure

- Promotes healthy stress response

Research Side Effects

- Redness, itchiness, and swelling of injection sites

- Nausea

- Flushing

- Do not use with other PDE-5 inhibitors (Sildenafil, Vardenafil, Tadalafil, Avanafil)

- Use with other PDE-5 can lead to priapism (too long and painful erection)

Matthew's Personal Insight on Research Cycling & Dosing

- The typical dosage is around 1 mg but can be increased up to 4 mg

- Best taken 45-60 minutes before intercourse

- One dose per 24 hours at the most. More can lead to desensitization of receptors.

- Effects can last up to 24-72 hours

Peptides & Supplements Matthew Would Stack With

- Any GHRH (Tesamorelin, MOD-GRF, Sermorelin, CJC-1295)

- Any GHRP (GHRP-2, GHRP-6, Ipamorelin, Hexarelin)

- Oxytocin

- VIP

- Kisspeptin-10

- Masculine Medicine

Pros & Cons

Pros

- Helps with sexual dysfunction in women and erectile dysfunction in men

- Works on the central nervous system

- It can be given through an intranasal spray

Cons

- Some feel the effects hours after using

- Can become dependent on sexual arousal without working on the root cause

Matthew's Opinion

- This is an all-around significant peptide to enhance a sex life

- I like how it works on the nervous system and can be used with both a man and a woman

- It is essential not to become dependent on this peptide.

- I would use it 1x week since the effects can last up to 72 hours.

9. Intro To Peptide Combo's

Disclaimer

This is how I currently approach all my peptide research. Except for the foregoing disclaimers, when referring to "you," I am referring to myself, as this is how I created the notes for my research techniques. Matthew Farrahi is not a doctor or qualified/accredited healthcare professional. The information displayed in these chapters is strictly for research and informational purposes and is neither intended to be medical advice/opinion nor should be considered as such. You should consult a qualified healthcare professional or doctor with any medical concerns, queries, or questions that you may have. Matthew Farrahi is a researcher, and any experiments or suggestions referred to in these chapters are designed solely for him. Any reader should not attempt, recreate, replicate, or explore them.

Why Combine Peptides

- Some peptides are best taken alone, and some can have a synergistic effect when combined.

- This is one of the aspects I hope to educate you on in this book so you have a better idea of which types of peptides work well together and which do not.

- For example, a category of peptides is called GHRH (Growth Hormone Releasing Hormone). These peptides help create growth hormone but do not release it. There is a category of peptides called GHRP (Growth Hormone Release Peptides). These peptides help release growth hormone.

- So, combining a GHRH with a GHRP would result in a synergistic effect

- Combining a GHRH with another GHRH would not result in a synergistic effect

When To Combine Peptides

- This comes down to goals, experience, and budget with peptides. Every peptide added to a cycle will increase the cost.

- And some peptides do not work well with some subjects. So, if a peptide blend is taken and the subject has an adverse reaction, it can be hard to tell which peptide it is.

- I recommend starting slowly in the peptide field to gain experience and see the response. As you gain experience, you can start looking into other peptides

Disclaimer About My Peptide Combinations

- This is part of the book where I share my opinions on peptides and what I would do. Tell you all the fun stuff that many people will not share.

- Many of them I have not tried. These are all blends I have either tried or have plans to try out

- It is essential to know that I am not a doctor; this is not medical advice.

- These are my experiments.

How To Use Peptide Combos?

- Pick one area to focus on

- Do not use multiple peptide combos at a time until one has gained experience

- Some combos will be repeated. Each combo can be used differently, and many have several benefits.

- The combos are organized from beginner to advanced.

- I have mentioned all the side effects for each peptide and peptide combo

- Side effects from peptides will never come close to side effects from pharmaceutical drugs, and most, if not all, can be prevented with conservative dosing and cycling

- That being said, being aware of the side effects is essential. Whether it's peptides, protein powder, a simple food, or a pharmaceutical drug, it is possible to experience side effects. I do my best to share what I would do to handle each peptide and peptide combo in the safest and most effective way.

10. Peptides Combos for Fat Loss

MOD-GRF-1295 + Ipamorelin

Overview

- MOD-GRF-1-29 is a GHRH (Growth Hormone Releasing Hormone)

- Ipamorelin is the mildest of GHRP's (Growth Hormone Releasing Peptide)

- This is one of the most commonly stacked GH peptides

Why Add These Together?

- MOD-GRF-1-29 goes up to the anterior pituitary gland and signals the body to create growth hormone

- Ipamorelin works by inhibiting somatostatin on the hypothalamus to allow the release of growth hormone.

- Combining these peptides ensures that the creation and release of growth hormones occur simultaneously.

Research Benefits

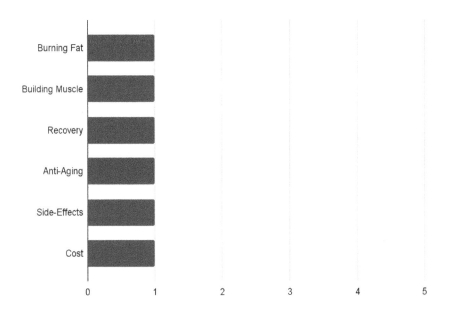

- Increase the creation and release of endogenous growth hormone

- Promotes muscle growth

- Helps with mood and stress resilience

- Slows down aging

- Improves sleep

- Promotes a balanced inflammatory response

- Improves bone density

Research Side Effects

- Redness, itchiness, and swelling of injection sites

- Water retention

- Facial flushing

Matthew's Personal Insight on Cycling & Dosing

- MOD-GRF-1-29

  - 100 mcg per injection (more is not better)

- Ipamorelin

  - 100-300 mcg per injection

  - Multiple injections can be given a day to increase GH secretion. Often used in bodybuilding

  - 5 days on, 2 days off, 10-12 weeks on, 4-8 weeks off

  - Carbohydrates and fatty acids can blunt growth hormone release. Best taken 30 minutes before eating or 2 hours after eating

Matthew's Personal Insight on Timing & Benefits

- Burning Fat

  - Before a workout in a fasted state

- Building Muscle

  - After a workout in a fasted state

- Sleep

  - Before bed in a fasted state

- General Anti-Aging

  - In the morning in a fasted state

Matthew's Opinion

- This is one of my favorite peptide combos that I have used for several years on and off

- Both of these peptides are well-used and well-researched and offer a wide ray of benefits

- I recommend most peptide beginners to look into this combo to get their feet wet with peptides before advancing

MOD-GRF-1295 + Ipamorelin + AOD-9604

Overview

- MOD-GRF-1-29 is a GHRH (Growth Hormone Releasing Hormone)

- Ipamorelin is the mildest of GHRP's (Growth Hormone Releasing Peptide)

- Anti-Obesity Drug-9604 (AOD-9604) is a synthetic fragment of the growth hormone amino acid

Why Add These Together?

- MOD-GRF-1-29 goes up to the anterior pituitary gland and signals the body to create and release growth hormone

- Ipamorelin works by inhibiting somatostatin on the hypothalamus to allow the release of growth hormone

- AOD-9604 does not use the hGH receptor on the pituitary gland, as it acts independently of that. This makes it a powerful peptide to stack with other GH peptides

- Combining these peptides ensures the creation and release of growth hormone occurs simultaneously while adding additional fat-burning benefits

Research Benefits

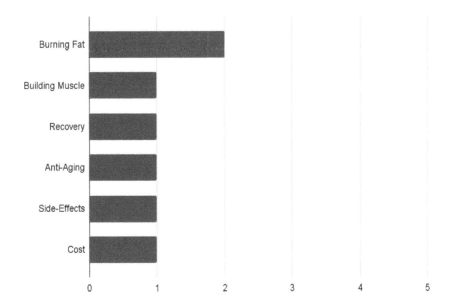

- Increase the creation and release of endogenous growth hormone

- Promotes muscle growth

- It helps regulate fat metabolism by stimulating lipolysis (breakdown of fat) and inhibiting lipogenesis (transformation of food into body fat

- Slows down aging

- Improves sleep

- Improves bone density

Research Side Effects

- Redness, itchiness, and swelling of injection sites

- Water retention

- Facial flushing

Matthew's Personal Insight on Cycling & Dosing

- MOD-GRF-1-29

  - ¤ 100 mcg per injection (more is not better)

- Ipamorelin

  - ¤ 100-300 mcg per injection

- AOD-9604

  - ¤ 250-300 mcg, 1-2x daily through a subcutaneous injection

- Multiple injections can be given a day to increase GH secretion. Often used in bodybuilding

- Carbohydrates and fatty acids can blunt growth hormone release. Best taken 30 minutes before eating and/or 2 hours after eating

- 5 days on, 2 days off, 10-12 weeks on, 4-8 weeks off

Matthew's Personal Insight on Timing & Benefits

- Burning Fat

  - ¤ Before a workout in a fasted state

- Building Muscle

  - ¤ After a workout in a fasted state

- Sleep

  - ¤ Before bed in a fasted state

- General Anti-Aging

  - ¤ In the morning in a fasted state

Matthew's Opinion

- This is another one of my favorite peptide combos that I have used for several years on and off

- All of these peptides have a wide ray of benefits with a high safety profile

- I like taking this peptide blend before a fasted workout

MOD-GRF-1295 + Ipamorelin + AOD-9604 + Semaglutide

Overview

- MOD-GRF-1-29 is a GHRH (Growth Hormone Releasing Hormone)

- Ipamorelin is the mildest of GHRPs (Growth Hormone Releasing Peptide)

- Anti-Obesity Drug-9604 (AOD-9604) is a synthetic fragment of the growth hormone amino acid

- Semaglutide is an FDA-approved medication for type-2 diabetes that possesses fat-burning properties

Why Add These Together?

- MOD-GRF-1-29 goes up to the anterior pituitary gland and signals the body to create growth hormone

- Ipamorelin works by inhibiting somatostatin on the hypothalamus to allow the release of growth hormone

- AOD-9604 does not use the hGH receptor on the pituitary gland, as it acts independently of that. This makes it a powerful peptide to stack with other GH peptides

- Semaglutide mimics the GLP-1 hormone released in the gut in response to eating

- Combining these peptides ensures the creation and release of growth hormone occurs simultaneously while adding additional fat-burning benefits and appetite control

Research Benefits

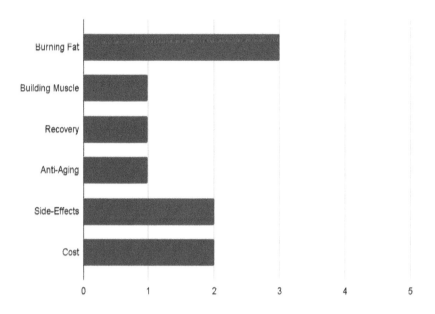

- Increase the creation and release of endogenous growth hormone

- Promotes muscle growth

- It helps regulate fat metabolism by stimulating lipolysis (breakdown of fat) and inhibiting lipogenesis (transformation of food into body fat)

- Slows down aging

- Improves sleep

- Improves bone density

- Manages appetite

Research Side Effects

- Redness, itchiness, and swelling of injection sites

- Water retention

- Facial flushing

- Abdominal pain

- Constipation

- Loss of appetite

- Hypoglycemia

Matthew's Personal Insight on Dosing

- MOD-GRF-1-29

  - 100 mcg per injection (more is not better)

- Ipamorelin

  - 100-300 mcg per injection

- AOD-9604

  - 250-300 mcg, 1-2x through a subcutaneous injection

- Semaglutide

  - 250 mcg, 1x a week for the first 4 weeks

  - Increasing the dose 250 mcg every 4 weeks

  - Do not exceed 2400 mcg per dose

Matthew's Personal Insight on Cycling

- MOD-GRF-1-29, Ipamorelin, AOD-9604

- ¤ Multiple GH peptides and AOD-9604 injections can be given daily to increase GH secretion and fat-burning benefits. Often used in bodybuilding

- ¤ Carbohydrates and fatty acids can blunt growth hormone release. Best taken 30 minutes before eating or 2 hours after eating

- ¤ 5 days on, 2 days off, 10-12 weeks on, 4-8 weeks off

- Semaglutide

  - ¤ 1x week, 2-3 months on, 2-3 months off

Matthew's Opinion

- MOD-GRF, Ipamorelin, and AOD-9604 is one of my favorite peptide combos that I have used for several years on and off

- Semaglutide is a great peptide to manage weight and appetite

- Semaglutide can be expensive, and I have encountered several having side-effects due to not eating enough food

- It is important to monitor nutrition levels when taking Semaglutide since many can go extended periods of not eating due to the appetite suppression the peptide offers

MOD-GRF-1295 + Ipamorelin + AOD-9604 + Tirezepatide

Overview

- MOD-GRF-1-29 is a GHRH (Growth Hormone Releasing Hormone)

- Ipamorelin is the mildest of GHRPs (Growth Hormone Releasing Peptide)

- Anti-Obesity Drug-9604 (AOD-9604) is a synthetic fragment of the growth hormone amino acid

- Tirezepatide is a synthetic modification of the glucose-dependent insulinotropic peptide (GIP)

Why Add These Together?

- MOD-GRF-1-29 goes up to the anterior pituitary gland and signals the body to create growth hormone

- Ipamorelin works by inhibiting somatostatin on the hypothalamus to allow the release of growth hormone

- AOD-9604 does not use the hGH receptor on the pituitary gland, as it acts independently of that. This makes it a powerful peptide to stack with other GH peptides

- Tirezepatide works both on GLP-1 and GIP receptors, which plays a major role in appetite control, regulating blood sugar, and enhancing metabolism

- Combining these peptides ensures growth hormone creation and release occurs simultaneously while adding additional fat-burning benefits and appetite control.

Research Benefits

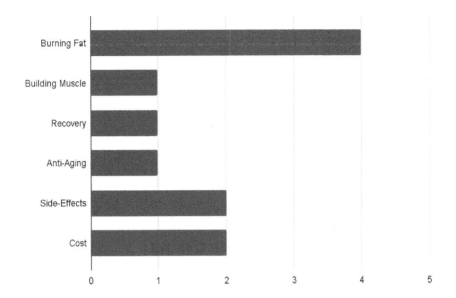

- Increase the creation and release of endogenous growth hormone

- Promotes muscle growth

- It helps regulate fat metabolism by stimulating lipolysis (breakdown of fat) and inhibiting lipogenesis (transformation of food into body fat

- Slows down aging

- Improves sleep

- Improves bone density

- Manages appetite

- Lowers blood sugar levels

Research Side Effects

- Redness, itchiness, and swelling of injection sites

- Water retention

- Facial flushing

- Abdominal pain

- Constipation

- Loss of appetite

- Hypoglycemia

Matthew's Personal Insight on Dosing

- MOD-GRF-1-29

  ¤ 100 mcg per injection (more is not better)

- Ipamorelin

  ¤ 100-300 mcg per injection

- AOD-9604

  ¤ 250-300 mcg per injection

- Tirezepatide

  ¤ 2.5 mg, 1x a week for the first 4 weeks

  ¤ 5 mg, 1x a week for the second 4 weeks

Matthew's Personal Insight on Cycling

- Ipamorelin, MOD-GRF-129, AOD-9604

  - ¤ Multiple GH peptides and AOD-9604 injections can be given daily to increase GH secretion and fat-burning benefits. Often used in bodybuilding

  - ¤ Carbohydrates and fatty acids can blunt growth hormone release. Best taken 30 minutes before eating or 2 hours after eating

  - ¤ 5 days on, 2 days off, 10-12 weeks on, 4-8 weeks off

- Tirezepatide

  - ¤ 1x week, 2-3 months on, 2-3 months off

Matthew's Personal Insight on Timing & Benefits

- Burning Fat

  - ¤ Before a workout in a fasted state

  - ¤ Best to take Tirzepatide in the morning in a fasted state

- Building Muscle (Not for Tirzepatide)

  - ¤ After a workout in a fasted state

- General Anti-Aging

  - ¤ In the morning in a fasted state

Matthew's Opinion

- MOD-GRF, Ipamorelin, and AOD-9604 is one of my favorite peptide combos that I have used for several years on and off

- Tirezepatide is a great peptide to manage weight and appetite. It would be my go-to weight-loss peptide

- Tirezepatide can be expensive, and I have encountered several having side effects due to not eating enough food

- It is important to monitor nutrition levels when taking Tirezepatide since many can go extended periods of not eating due to the appetite suppression the peptide offers

Tesamorelin + Ipamorelin + AOD-9604 + Semaglutide

Overview

- Tesamorelin is a GHRH (Growth Hormone Releasing Hormone)

- Ipamorelin is the mildest of GHRP's (Growth Hormone Releasing Peptide)

- Anti-Obesity Drug-9604 (AOD-9604) is a synthetic fragment of the growth hormone amino acid

- Semaglutide is an FDA-approved medication for type-2 diabetes that possesses fat-burning properties

Why Add These Together?

- Tesamorelin goes up to the anterior pituitary gland and signals the body to create growth hormone (Stronger than MOD-GRF-1-29)

- Ipamorelin works by inhibiting somatostatin on the hypothalamus to allow the release of growth hormone

- AOD-9604 does not use the hGH receptor on the pituitary gland, as it acts independently of that. This makes it a powerful peptide to stack with other GH peptides

- Semaglutide mimics the GLP-1 hormone released in the gut in response to eating

- Combining these peptides ensures the creation and release of growth hormone occurs simultaneously while adding additional fat-burning benefits and appetite control

Research Benefits

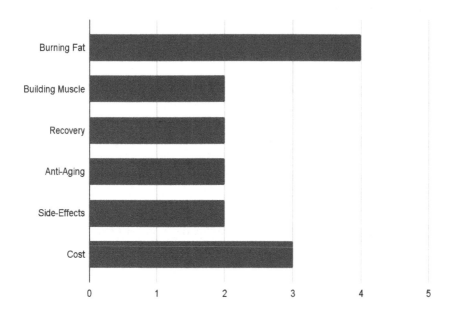

- Increase the creation and release of endogenous growth hormone

- Promotes muscle growth

- It helps regulate fat metabolism by stimulating lipolysis (breakdown of fat) and inhibiting lipogenesis (transformation of food into body fat

- Slows down aging

- Improves sleep

- Improves bone density

- Manages appetite

Research Side Effects

- Redness, itchiness, and swelling of injection sites

- Water retention

- Facial flushing

- Abdominal pain

- Constipation

- Loss of appetite

- Hypoglycemia

- Sharp increase in IGF-1 levels

Matthew's Personal Insight on Dosing

- Tesamorelin

  ¤ 500-2000 mcg per injection

- Ipamorelin

  ¤ 100-300 mcg per injection

- AOD-9604

  ¤ 250-300 mcg, 1-2x through a subcutaneous injection

- Semaglutide

  ¤ 250 mcg, 1x a week for the first 4 weeks

  ¤ Increasing the dose 250 mcg every 4 weeks

  ¤ Do not exceed 2400 mcg per dose

Matthew's Personal Insight on Cycling

- Tesamorelin, Ipamorelin, AOD-9604

- ¤ Multiple GH peptides and AOD-9604 injections can be given daily to increase GH secretion and fat-burning benefits. Often used in bodybuilding

- ¤ Carbohydrates and fatty acids can blunt growth hormone release. Best taken 30 minutes before eating or 2 hours after eating

- ¤ 5 days on, 2 days off, 10-12 weeks on, 4-8 weeks off

- Semaglutide

  - ¤ 1x week, 2-3 months on, 2-3 months off

Matthew's Personal Insight on Timing & Benefits

- Burning Fat

  - ¤ Before a workout in a fasted state

  - ¤ Best to take Semaglutide in the morning in a fasted state

- Building Muscle (Not for Semaglutide)

  - ¤ After a workout in a fasted state

- General Anti-Aging

  - ¤ In the morning in a fasted state

Matthew's Opinion

- Tesamorelin, Ipamorelin and AOD-9604 is one of my favorite peptide combos

- Tesamorelin is an excellent upgrade replacement from MOD-GRF-1-29. I would start at a more conservative dosing and cycling scheme and work up as I got more comfortable

- Semaglutide is a great peptide to manage weight and appetite

- Semaglutide can be expensive, and I have encountered several having side-effects due to not eating enough food

- It is important to monitor nutrition levels when taking Semaglutide since many can go extended periods of not eating due to the appetite suppression the peptide offers

Tesamorelin + Ipamorelin + AOD-9604 + Tirezepatide

Overview

- Tesamorelin is a GHRH (Growth Hormone Releasing Hormone)

- Ipamorelin is the mildest of GHRP's (Growth Hormone Releasing Peptide)

- Anti-Obesity Drug-9604 (AOD-9604) is a synthetic fragment of the growth hormone amino acid

- Tirezepatide is a synthetic modification of the glucose-dependent insulinotropic peptide (GIP)

Why Add These Together?

- Tesamorelin goes up to the anterior pituitary gland and signals the body to create growth hormone (Stronger than MOD-GRF-1-29)

- Ipamorelin works by inhibiting somatostatin on the hypothalamus to allow the release of growth hormone

- AOD-9604 does not use the hGH receptor on the pituitary gland, as it acts independently of that. This makes it a powerful peptide to stack with other GH peptides

- Tirezepatide works both on GLP-1 and GIP receptors, which plays a major role in appetite control, regulating blood sugar, and enhancing metabolism

- Combining these peptides ensures the creation and release of growth hormone occurs simultaneously while adding additional fat-burning benefits and appetite control

Research Benefits

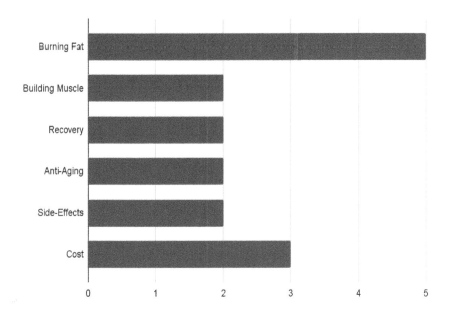

- Increase the creation and release of endogenous growth hormone

- Promotes muscle growth

- It helps regulate fat metabolism by stimulating lipolysis (breakdown of fat) and inhibiting lipogenesis (transformation of food into body fat

- Slows down aging

- Improves sleep

- Improves bone density

- Manages appetite

- Lowers blood sugar levels

Research Side Effects

- Redness, itchiness, and swelling of injection sites

- Water retention

- Facial flushing

- Abdominal pain

- Constipation

- Loss of appetite

- Hypoglycemia

- Sharp increase in IGF-1 levels

Matthew's Personal Insight on Dosing

- Tesamorelin

  - 500-2000 mcg per injection

- Ipamorelin

  - 100-300 mcg per injection

- AOD-9604

  - 250-300 mcg per injection

- Tirezepatide

  - 2.5 mg, 1x a week for the first 4 weeks

  - 5 mg, 1x a week for the second 4 weeks

Matthew's Personal Insight on Cycling

- Ipamorelin, Tesamorelin, AOD-9604

- ¤ Multiple GH peptides and AOD-9604 injections can be given daily to increase GH secretion and fat-burning benefits. Often used in bodybuilding

- ¤ Carbohydrates and fatty acids can blunt growth hormone release. Best taken 30 minutes before eating or 2 hours after eating

- ¤ 5 days on, 2 days off, 10-12 weeks on, 4-8 weeks off

- Tirezepatide

- ¤ 1x week, 2-3 months on, 2-3 months off

Matthew's Personal Insight on Timing & Benefits

- Burning Fat

- ¤ Before a workout in a fasted state

- ¤ Best to take Tirezepatide in the morning in a fasted state

- Building Muscle (Not for Tirezepatide)

- ¤ After a workout in a fasted state

- General Anti-Aging

- ¤ In the morning in a fasted state

Matthew's Opinion

- Tesamorelin, Ipamorelin, and AOD-9604 is one of my favorite peptide combos.

- Tesamorelin is a nice upgrade replacement from MOD-GRF-1-29. I would start with a more conservative dosing scheme and increase as I got more comfortable

- Tirezepatide is a great peptide to manage weight and appetite. It would be my go-to weight-loss peptide

- Tirezepatide can be expensive, and I have encountered several having side effects due to not eating enough food

- It is important to monitor nutrition levels when taking Tirezepatide since many can go extended periods of not eating due to the appetite suppression the peptide offers

Tesamorelin + Ipamorelin + AOD-9604 + Tirezepatide + 5 Amino-1-MQ

Overview

- Tesamorelin is a GHRH (Growth Hormone Releasing Hormone)

- Ipamorelin is the mildest of GHRPs (Growth Hormone Releasing Peptide)

- Anti-Obesity Drug-9604 (AOD-9604) is a synthetic fragment of the growth hormone amino acid

- Tirezepatide is a synthetic modification of the glucose-dependent insulinotropic peptide (GIP)

- 5-Amino-1-MQ is an oral peptide that is most commonly used to help reduce fat

Why Add These Together?

- Tesamorelin goes up to the anterior pituitary gland and signals the body to create growth hormone (Stronger than MOD-GRF-1-29)

- Ipamorelin works by inhibiting somatostatin on the hypothalamus to allow the release of growth hormone

- AOD-9604 does not use the hGH receptor on the pituitary gland, as it acts independently of that. This makes it a powerful peptide to stack with other GH peptides

- Tirezepatide works both on GLP-1 and GIP receptors, which plays a major role in appetite control, regulating blood sugar, and enhancing metabolism

- 5-Amino-1-MQ blocks the activity of NNMT. This creates an increase in NAD+, which is crucial for a wide array of cellular processes, one being the metabolic rate

- Combining these peptides ensures the creation and release of growth hormone occur simultaneously while adding additional fat-burning benefits, appetite control, and enhanced cellular functions from the increase in NAD+

Research Benefits

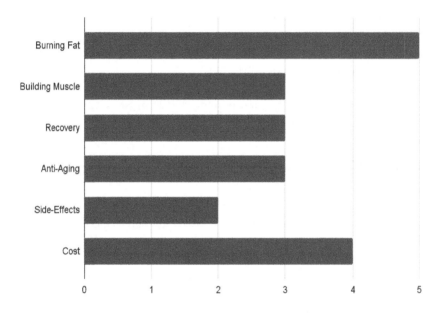

- Increase the creation and release of endogenous growth hormone

- Promotes muscle growth

- It helps regulate fat metabolism by stimulating lipolysis (breakdown of fat) and inhibiting lipogenesis (transformation of food into body fat)

- Slows down aging

- Improves sleep

- Improves bone density

- Manages appetite

- Lowers blood sugar levels

- Improves energy levels

Research Side Effects

- Redness, itchiness, and swelling of injection sites

- Water retention

- Facial flushing

- Abdominal pain

- Constipation

- Loss of appetite

- Hypoglycemia

- Sharp increase in IGF-1 levels

Matthew's Personal Insight on Dosing

- Tesamorelin

  - 500-2000 mcg per injection

- Ipamorelin

  - 100-300 mcg per injection

- AOD-9604

  - 250-300 mcg per injection

- 5-Amino-1-MQ

  - ¤ 50-150 mg, taken all at once or split up

- Tirezepatide

  - ¤ 2.5 mg, 1x a week for the first 4 weeks

  - ¤ 5mg, 1x a week for the second 4 weeks

Matthew's Personal Insight on Cycling

- Ipamorelin, Tesamorelin, AOD-9604

  - ¤ Multiple GH peptides and AOD-9604 injections can be given daily to increase GH secretion and fat-burning benefits. Often used in bodybuilding

  - ¤ Carbohydrates and fatty acids can blunt growth hormone release. Best taken 30 minutes before eating or 2 hours after eating

  - ¤ 5 days on, 2 days off, 10-12 weeks on, 4-8 weeks off

- Tirezepatide

  - ¤ 1x week, 2-3 months on, 2-3 months off

- 5-Amino-1-MQ

  - ¤ It is important to take with food due to 5-Amino-1-MQ being oil-solubility

  - ¤ It is ideal to take it in the morning to prevent sleep disturbances

  - ¤ 3-6 weeks on, 1-3 weeks off

Matthew's Personal Insight on Timing & Benefits

- Burning Fat

  - Before a workout in a fasted state (except for 5-Amino-1-MQ, take with food)

  - Best to take Tirezepatide in the morning in a fasted state

- Building Muscle (Not for Tirezepatide or 5-Amino-1-MQ)

  - After a workout in a fasted state

- General Anti-Aging

  - In the morning in a fasted state

Matthew's Opinion

- Tesamorelin, Ipamorelin, and AOD-9604 are one of my favorite peptide combos

- Tesamorelin is an excellent upgrade replacement from MOD-GRF-1-29. I would start at a more conservative dosing scheme and increase as I got more comfortable

- Tirezepatide is a great peptide to manage weight and appetite. It would be my go-to weight-loss peptide

- Tirezepatide can be expensive, and I have encountered several having side-effects due to not eating enough food

- It is important to monitor nutrition levels when taking Tirezepatide since many can go extended periods of not eating due to the appetite suppression the peptide offers

- 5-Amino-1-MQ is a great peptide, although expensive, to take due to the increase in NAD+, which seems promising to aid in multiple cellular processes

11. Peptides Combos for Building Muscle

MOD-GRF-1-29 + Ipamorelin

Overview

- MOD-GRF-1-29 is a GHRH (Growth Hormone Releasing Hormone)

- This is one of the most commonly stacked GH peptides

- Ipamorelin is the mildest of GHRPs (Growth Hormone Releasing Peptide)

Why Add These Together?

- MOD-GRF-1-29 goes up to the anterior pituitary gland and signals the body to create growth hormone

- Ipamorelin works by inhibiting somatostatin on the hypothalamus to allow the release of growth hormone

- Combining these peptides ensures the creation and release of growth hormone occurs simultaneously

Research Benefits

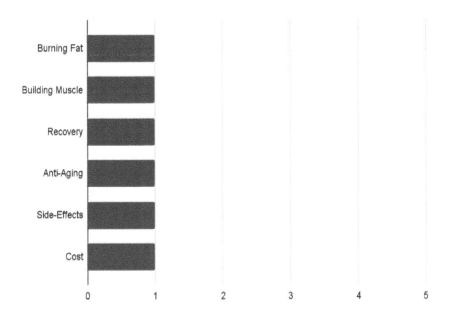

- Increase the creation and release of endogenous growth hormone

- Promotes muscle growth

- Helps with mood and stress resilience

- Slows down aging

- Improves sleep

- Promotes a balanced inflammatory response

- Improves bone density

Research Side Effects

- Redness, itchiness, and swelling of injection sites

- Water retention

- Facial flushing bone density

Matthew's Personal Insight on Research Dosing & Cycling

- MOD-GRF-1-29

  - 100 mcg per injection (more is not better)

- Ipamorelin

  - 100-300 mcg per injection

- Multiple injections can be given a day to increase GH secretion. Often used in bodybuilding

- 5 days on, 2 days off, 10-12 weeks on, 4-8 weeks off

- Carbohydrates and fatty acids can blunt growth hormone release. Best taken 30 minutes before eating or 2 hours after eating

Matthew's Personal Insight on Research Timing & Benefits

- Burning Fat

  - Before a workout in a fasted state

- Building Muscle

  - After a workout in a fasted state

- Sleep

  - Before bed in a fasted state

- General Anti-Aging

  - In the morning in a fasted state

Matthew's Opinion

- This is one of my favorite peptide combos that I have used for several years on and off

- Both of these peptides are well-used and well-researched and offer a wide ray of benefits

- I recommend most peptide beginners to look into this combo to get their feet wet with peptides before advancing

MOD-GRF-1295 + GHRP-6

Overview

- MOD-GRF-1-29 is a GHRH (Growth Hormone Releasing Hormone)

- GHRP-6 is the third strongest GHRP (Growth Hormone Releasing Peptide)

Why Add These Together?

- MOD-GRF-1-29 goes up to the anterior pituitary gland and signals the body to create growth hormone

- GHRP-6 works by inhibiting somatostatin on the hypothalamus to allow the release of growth hormone

- Combining these peptides ensures the creation and release of growth hormone occurs simultaneously

- GHRP-6 increases hunger, making this a great combo if bulking is a main focus

Research Benefits

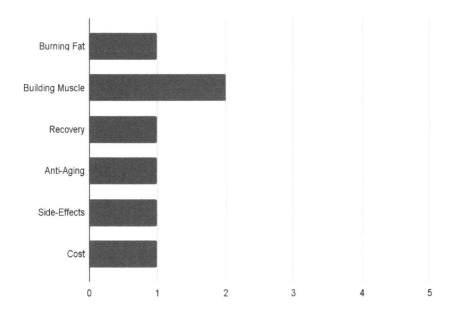

- Increase the creation and release of endogenous growth hormone

- Promotes muscle growth

- Helps with mood and stress resilience

- Slows down aging

- Improves sleep

- Promotes a balanced inflammatory response

- Improves bone density

Research Side Effects

- Redness, itchiness, and swelling of injection sites

- Water retention

- Facial flushing

- Stimulates ghrelin

- Increases in stress responses through an increase in prolactin, ACTH, and cortisol

Matthew's Personal Insight on Research Dosing & Cycling

- MOD-GRF-1-29

  - ¤ 100 mcg per injection (more is not better)

- GHRP-6

  - ¤ 100 mcg per injection

- Multiple injections can be given a day to increase GH secretion. Often used in bodybuilding

- 5 days on, 2 days off, 10-12 weeks on, 4-8 weeks off

- Carbohydrates and fatty acids can blunt growth hormone release. Best taken 30 minutes before eating or 2 hours after eating

Matthew's Personal Insight on Research Timing & Benefits

- Burning Fat

  - ¤ Before a workout in a fasted state

- Building Muscle

  - ¤ After a workout in a fasted state

- Sleep

  - ¤ Before bed in a fasted state

- General Anti-Aging

  - ⌑ In the morning in a fasted state

Matthew's Opinion

- This would be one of the beginner peptide combos I would use if I wanted to focus on bulking.

- I like how GHRP-6 stimulates hunger with fewer side effects than GHRP-2

- I would switch out GHRP-6 with Ipamorelin throughout the week (3 days GHRP-6, 2 days Ipamorelin) to monitor bulk unless trying to do a massive bulk

MOD-GRF-129 + GHRP-2

Overview

- MOD-GRF-1-29 is a GHRH (Growth Hormone Releasing Hormone)

- GHRP-2 is the second strongest GHRP (Growth Hormone Releasing Peptide)

Why Add These Together?

- MOD-GRF-1-29 goes up to the anterior pituitary gland and signals the body to create growth hormone

- GHRP-2 works by inhibiting somatostatin on the hypothalamus to allow the release of growth hormone

- Combining these peptides ensures the creation and release of growth hormone occurs simultaneously

- GHRP-2 increases hunger and has a stronger release of growth hormone than GHRP-2 and Ipamorelin, making this a powerful combo for muscle-building

Research Benefits

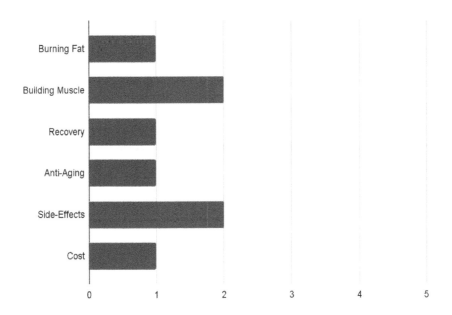

- Increase the creation and release of endogenous growth hormone

- Promotes muscle growth

- Helps with mood and stress resilience

- Slows down aging

- Improves sleep

- Promotes a balanced inflammatory response

- Improves bone density

Research Side Effects

- Redness, itchiness, and swelling of injection sites

- Water retention

- Facial flushing

- Stimulates ghrelin (less than GHRP-6)

- Prolonged use and over-saturation of receptors may increase anxiety and depression

- Increases in stress responses through an increase in prolactin, ACTH, and cortisol

Matthew's Personal Insight on Research Dosing & Cycling

- MOD-GRF-1-29

  - 100 mcg per injection (more is not better)

- GHRP-2

  - 100 mcg per injection

- Multiple injections can be given a day to increase GH secretion. Often used in bodybuilding

- 5 days on, 2 days off, 10-12 weeks on, 4-8 weeks off

- Carbohydrates and fatty acids can blunt growth hormone release. Best taken 30 minutes before eating or 2 hours after eating

Matthew's Personal Insight on Research Timing & Benefits

- Burning Fat

  - Before a workout in a fasted state

- Building Muscle

  - After a workout in a fasted state

- Sleep

    ⌷ Before bed in a fasted state

- General Anti-Aging

    ⌷ In the morning in a fasted state

Matthew's Opinion

- It is important to monitor closely when using GHRP-2 since prolonged use can lead to more side effects

- I would stick to shorter cycles when using GHRP-2 since it is a stronger GHRP and has more side effects compared to Ipamorelin

- I would switch out GHRP-2 with Ipamorelin throughout the week (3 days GHRP-2, 2 days Ipamorelin) to still get the stronger growth hormone release while reducing the unwanted side-effects that may happen from GHRP-2

MOD-GRF-1295 + GHRP-6 + BPC-157

Overview

- MOD-GRF-1-29 is a GHRH (Growth Hormone Releasing Hormone)

- GHRP-6 is the third strongest GHRP (Growth Hormone Releasing Peptide)

- BPC-157 stands for body-protective compound. It was discovered in the human gastric juice

Why Add These Together?

- MOD-GRF-1-29 goes up to the anterior pituitary gland and signals the body to create growth hormone

- GHRP-6 works by inhibiting somatostatin on the hypothalamus to allow the release of growth hormone

- GHRP-6 increases hunger, making this a great addition if bulking is the main focus

- BPC-157 enhances growth hormone absorption while adding neuroprotective (brain), cardioprotective (heart), gastroprotective (stomach), and musculoskeletal protective (joints, ligaments and muscles) benefits

- Combining these peptides ensures the creation and release of growth hormone occur simultaneously while adding enhanced growth hormone absorption and full body recovery

Research Benefits

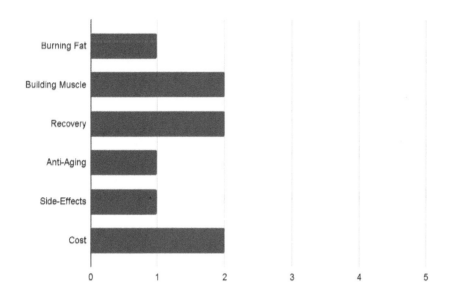

- Increase the creation and release of endogenous growth hormone

- Promotes muscle growth

- Helps with mood and stress resilience

- Slows down aging

- Neuroprotective (brain), cardioprotective (heart), gastroprotective (stomach), and musculoskeletal protective (joints, ligaments and muscles)

- Improves sleep

- Promotes a balanced inflammatory response

- Improves bone density

Research Side Effects

- Redness, itchiness, and swelling of injection sites

- Water retention

- Facial flushing

- Stimulates ghrelin

- Increases in stress responses through increase in prolactin, ACTH and cortisol

Matthew's Personal Insight on Research Dosing

- MOD-GRF-1-29

  ⌑ 100 mcg per injection (more is not better)

- GHRP-6

  ⌑ 100 mcg per injection

- BPC-157

  ⌑ 300-600 mcg per injection

  ⌑ For an injury: Split dose into 200-300 mcg and inject around the area

Matthew's Personal Insight on Research Cycling

- MOD-GRF-1-29, GHRP-6

  ⌑ Multiple injections can be given a day to increase GH secretion. Often used in bodybuilding

  ⌑ Carbohydrates and fatty acids can blunt growth hormone release. Best taken 30 minutes before eating and/or 2 hours after eating

- 5 days on, 2 days off, 10-12 weeks on, 4-8 weeks off
- BPC-157
  - 5 days on, 2 days off, 10-12 weeks on, 4-8 weeks off
  - It can be cycled continuously
  - Best to take when the body needs recovery (post-workout, recovery days, before bed)

Matthew's Personal Insight on Research Timing & Benefits

- Burning Fat
  - Before a workout in a fasted state
- Building Muscle
  - After a workout in a fasted state
  - Best time to take BPC-157
- Sleep
  - Before bed in a fasted state
- General Anti-Aging
  - In the morning in a fasted state

Matthew's Opinion

- This is an awesome peptide muscle-building combo that I plan to use myself
- I like how GHRP-6 stimulates hunger with fewer side effects than GHRP-2

- I like how BPC-157 enhances the recovery aspect, leading to better gains and enhancing growth hormone absorption

- I would switch out GHRP-6 with Ipamorelin throughout the week (3 days GHRP-6, 2 days Ipamorelin) to monitor bulk unless trying to do a massive bulk

MOD-GRF-1295 + GHRP-2 + BPC-157

Overview

- MOD-GRF-1-29 is a GHRH (Growth Hormone Releasing Hormone)

- GHRP-2 is the second strongest GHRP (Growth Hormone Releasing Peptide)

- BPC-157 stands for body-protective compound. It was discovered in the human gastric juice

Why Add These Together?

- MOD-GRF-1-29 goes up to the anterior pituitary gland and signals the body to create growth hormone

- GHRP-2 works by inhibiting somatostatin on the hypothalamus to allow the release of growth hormone

- GHRP-2 increases hunger and has a stronger release of growth hormone than GHRP-6 and Ipamorelin, making this a powerful combo for muscle-building

- BPC-157 enhances growth hormone absorption while adding neuroprotective (brain), cardioprotective (heart), gastroprotective (stomach), and musculoskeletal protective (joints, ligaments and muscles) benefits

- Combining these peptides ensures the creation and release of growth hormone occur simultaneously while adding enhanced growth hormone absorption and full body recovery

Research Benefits

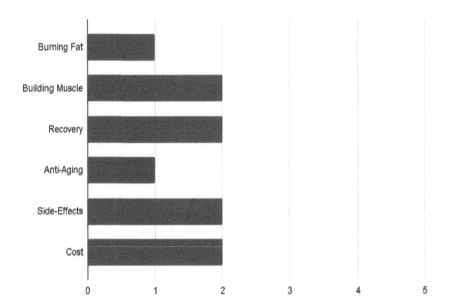

- Increase the creation and release of endogenous growth hormone

- Promotes muscle growth

- Helps with mood and stress resilience

- Slows down aging

- Neuroprotective (brain), cardioprotective (heart), gastroprotective (stomach), and musculoskeletal protective (joints, ligaments and muscles)

- Improves sleep

- Promotes a balanced inflammatory response

- Improves bone density

Research Side Effects

- Redness, itchiness, and swelling of injection sites

- Water retention

- Facial flushing

- Stimulates ghrelin

- Increases in stress responses through an increase in prolactin, ACTH, and cortisol

- Prolonged use and over-saturation of receptors may increase anxiety and depression

Matthew's Personal Insight on Research Dosing

- MOD-GRF-1-29

  - ¤ 100 mcg per injection (more is not better)

- GHRP-2

  - ¤ 100 mcg per injection

- BPC-157

  - ¤ 300-600 mcg per injection

  - ¤ For an injury: Split the dose into 200-300 mcg and inject around the area

Matthew's Personal Insight on Research Cycling

- MOD-GRF-1-29, GHRP-2

  - ¤ Multiple injections can be given a day to increase GH secretion. Often used in bodybuilding

- Carbohydrates and fatty acids can blunt growth hormone release. Best taken 30 minutes before eating or 2 hours after eating

- 5 days on, 2 days off, 10-12 weeks on, 4-8 weeks off

- BPC-157

  - 5 days on, 2 days off, 10-12 weeks on, 4-8 weeks off

  - It can be cycled continuously

  - Best to take when the body needs recovery (post-workout, recovery days, before bed)

Matthew's Personal Insight on Research Timing & Benefits

- Burning Fat

  - Before a workout in a fasted state

- Building Muscle

  - After a workout in a fasted state

  - Best time to take BPC-157

- Sleep

  - Before bed in a fasted state

- General Anti-Aging

  - In the morning in a fasted state

Matthew's Opinion

- I like how BPC-157 enhances the recovery aspect, leading to better gains and enhancing growth hormone absorption

- It is important to monitor closely when using GHRP-2, since prolonged use can lead to more side-effects

- I would stick to shorter cycles when using GHRP-2, since it is a stronger GHRP and has more side effects compared to Ipamorelin

- I would switch out GHRP-2 with Ipamorelin throughout the week (3 days GHRP-2, 2 days Ipamorelin) to still get the stronger growth hormone release while reducing the unwanted side-effects that may happen from GHRP-2.

MOD-GRF-1295 + GHRP-6 + BPC-157 + DSIP

Overview

- MOD-GRF-1-29 is a GHRH (Growth Hormone Releasing Hormone)

- GHRP-6 is the third strongest GHRP (Growth Hormone Releasing Peptide)

- BPC-157 stands for body-protective compound. It was discovered in the human gastric juice

- DSIP stands for Delta Sleep-Inducing Peptide

Why Add These Together?

- MOD-GRF-1-29 goes up to the anterior pituitary gland and signals the body to create growth hormone

- GHRP-6 works by inhibiting somatostatin on the hypothalamus to allow the release of growth hormone

- GHRP-6 increases hunger, making this a great addition if bulking is the main focus

- DSIP has been shown to increase endocrine functions during sleep, leading to higher releases of growth hormone, thyroid hormone, and testosterone. And DSIP helps aid in falling and staying asleep

- BPC-157 enhances growth hormone absorption while adding neuroprotective (brain), cardioprotective (heart), gastroprotective (stomach), and musculoskeletal protective (joints, ligaments and muscles) benefits

- Combining these peptides ensures the creation and release of growth hormone occur simultaneously while adding enhanced growth hormone absorption, full body recovery, and deeper sleep with larger releases of growth hormone and testosterone during sleep

Research Benefits

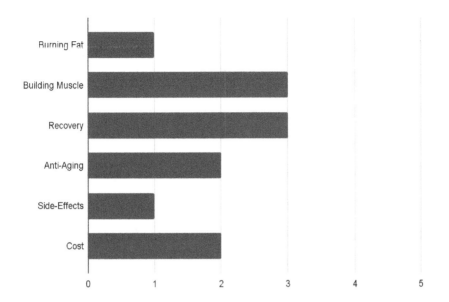

- Increase the creation and release of endogenous growth hormone

- Promotes muscle growth

- Helps with mood and stress resilience

- Slows down aging

- Neuroprotective (brain), cardioprotective (heart), gastroprotective (stomach), and musculoskeletal protective (joints, ligaments and muscles)

- Improves sleep quality

- Improves bone density

- Stimulates LH (Luteinizing Hormone) and GHRH (Growth Hormone Releasing Hormone)

Research Side Effects

- Redness, itchiness, and swelling of injection sites

- Water retention

- Facial flushing

- Stimulates ghrelin

- May disrupt sleep

- Increases in stress responses through an increase in prolactin, ACTH, and cortisol

Matthew's Personal Insight on Research Dosing

- MOD-GRF-1-29

  - 100 mcg per injection (more is not better)

- GHRP-6

  - 100 mcg per injection

- BPC-157

  - 300-600 mcg per injection

  - For an injury: Split the dose into 200-300 mcg and inject around the area

- DSIP

  - 100 mcg 3 hours before bed daily

  - Reduce down to 50 mcg 1x weekly once sleep stabilizes

Matthew's Personal Insight on Research Cycling

- MOD-GRF-1-29, GHRP-6

- ¤ Multiple injections can be given a day to increase GH secretion. Often used in bodybuilding

- ¤ Carbohydrates and fatty acids can blunt growth hormone release. Best taken 30 minutes before eating and/or 2 hours after eating

- ¤ 5 days on, 2 days off, 10-12 weeks on, 4-8 weeks off

- BPC-157

  - ¤ 5 days on, 2 days off, 10-12 weeks on, 4-8 weeks off

  - ¤ It can be cycled continuously

  - ¤ Best to take when the body needs recovery (post-workout, recovery days, before bed)

- DSIP

  - ¤ Only used until sleep stabilizes

  - ¤ Reduce dose and frequency as sleep improves

Matthew's Personal Insight on Research Timing & Benefits

- Burning Fat

  - ¤ Before a workout in a fasted state

- Building Muscle

  - ¤ After a workout in a fasted state

  - ¤ Best time to take BPC-157

- Sleep

  - ¤ Before bed in a fasted state

  - ¤ Only time to take DSIP - 3 hours before bed

- General Anti-Aging

  ¤ In the morning in a fasted state

Matthew's Opinion

- DSIP is a great peptide to add to this muscle-building protocol. It is fairly inexpensive, deepens sleep, and enhances growth hormone and testosterone secretion

- I like how GHRP-6 stimulates hunger with fewer side effects than GHRP-2

- I like how BPC-157 enhances the recovery aspect, leading to better gains and enhances growth hormone absorption

- I would switch out GHRP-6 with Ipamorelin throughout the week (3 days GHRP-6, 2 days Ipamorelin) to monitor bulk unless trying to do a massive bulk.

MOD-GRF-1295 + GHRP-2 + BPC-157 + DSIP

Overview

- MOD-GRF-1-29 is a GHRH (Growth Hormone Releasing Hormone)

- GHRP-2 is the second strongest GHRP (Growth Hormone Releasing Peptide)

- BPC-157 stands for body-protective compound. It was discovered in the human gastric juice

- DSIP stands for Delta Sleep-Inducing Peptide

Why Add These Together?

- MOD-GRF-1-29 goes up to the anterior pituitary gland and signals the body to create growth hormone

- GHRP-2 works by inhibiting somatostatin on the hypothalamus to allow the release of growth hormone

- GHRP-2 increases hunger and has a stronger release of growth hormone than GHRP-6 and Ipamorelin, making this a powerful combo for muscle-building

- DSIP has been shown to increase endocrine functions during sleep, leading to higher releases of growth hormone, thyroid hormone, and testosterone. And DSIP helps aid in falling and staying asleep

- BPC-157 enhances growth hormone absorption while adding neuroprotective (brain), cardioprotective (heart), gastroprotective (stomach), and musculoskeletal protective (joints, ligaments and muscles) benefits

- Combining these peptides ensures the creation and release of growth hormone occur simultaneously while adding enhanced growth hormone absorption, full body recovery, and deeper sleep with larger releases of growth hormone and testosterone during sleep

Research Benefits

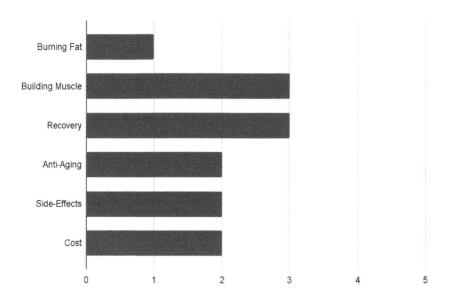

- Increase the creation and release of endogenous growth hormone

- Promotes muscle growth

- Helps with mood and stress resilience

- Slows down aging

- Neuroprotective (brain), cardioprotective (heart), gastroprotective (stomach), and musculoskeletal protective (joints, ligaments and muscles)

- Improves sleep quality

- Improves bone density

- Stimulates LH (Luteinizing Hormone) and GHRH (Growth Hormone Releasing Hormone)

Research Side Effects

- Redness, itchiness, and swelling of injection sites

- Water retention

- Facial flushing

- Stimulates ghrelin

- May disrupt sleep

- Increases in stress responses through an increase in prolactin, ACTH and cortisol

- Prolonged use and over-saturation of receptors may increase anxiety and depression

Matthew's Personal Insight on Research Dosing

- MOD-GRF-1-29

  - 100 mcg per injection (more is not better)

- GHRP-2

  - 100 mcg per injection

- BPC-157

  - 300-600 mcg per injection

  - For an injury: Split the dose into 200-300 mcg and inject around the area

- DSIP

  - 100 mcg 3 hours before bed daily

- ¤ Reduce down to 50 mcg 1x weekly once sleep stabilizes

Matthew's Personal Insight on Research Cycling

- MOD-GRF-1-29, GHRP-2

  - ¤ Multiple injections can be given a day to increase GH secretion. Often used in bodybuilding

  - ¤ Carbohydrates and fatty acids can blunt growth hormone release. Best taken 30 minutes before eating and/or 2 hours after eating

  - ¤ 5 days on, 2 days off, 10-12 weeks on, 4-8 weeks off

- BPC-157

  - ¤ 5 days on, 2 days off, 10-12 weeks on, 4-8 weeks off

  - ¤ It can be cycled continuously

  - ¤ Best to take when the body needs recovery (post-workout, recovery days, before bed)

- DSIP

  - ¤ Only used until sleep stabilizes

  - ¤ Reduce dose and frequency as sleep improves

Matthew's Personal Insight on Research Timing & Benefits

- Burning Fat

  - ¤ Before a workout in a fasted state

- Building Muscle

  - ¤ After a workout in a fasted state

- ¤ Best time to take BPC-157

- Sleep

  - ¤ Before bed in a fasted state

  - ¤ Only time to take DSIP - 3 hours before bed

- General Anti-Aging

  - ¤ In the morning in a fasted state

Matthew's Opinion

- DSIP is a great peptide to add to this muscle-building protocol. It is fairly inexpensive, deepens sleep, and enhances growth hormone and testosterone secretion

- It is important to monitor closely when using GHRP-2, since prolonged use can lead to more side-effects

- I would stick to shorter cycles when using GHRP-2, since it is a stronger GHRP and has more side effects compared to Ipamorelin & GHRP-6

- I like how BPC-157 enhances the recovery aspect, leading to better gains and enhancing growth hormone absorption

- I would switch out GHRP-2 with Ipamorelin throughout the week (3 days GHRP-2, 2 days Ipamorelin) to still get the stronger growth hormone release while reducing the unwanted side-effects that may happen from GHRP-

Tesamorelin + GHRP-6 + BPC-157

Overview

- Tesamorelin is a GHRH (Growth Hormone Releasing Hormone)

- GHRP-6 is the third strongest GHRP (Growth Hormone Releasing Peptide)

- BPC-157 stands for body-protective compound. It was discovered in the human gastric juice

Why Add These Together?

- Tesamorelin goes up to the anterior pituitary gland and signals the body to create growth hormone (Stronger than MOD-GRF-1-29)

- GHRP-6 works by inhibiting somatostatin on the hypothalamus to allow the release of growth hormone

- GHRP-6 increases hunger, making this a great addition if bulking is the main focus

- BPC-157 enhances growth hormone absorption while adding neuroprotective (brain), cardioprotective (heart), gastroprotective (stomach), and musculoskeletal protective (joints, ligaments and muscles) benefits

- Combining these peptides ensures the creation and release of growth hormone occurs simultaneously while adding enhance growth hormone absorption and full body recovery

Research Benefits

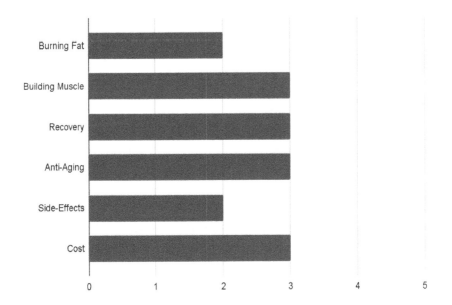

- Increase the creation and release of endogenous growth hormone

- Promotes muscle growth

- Helps with mood and stress resilience

- Slows down aging

- Neuroprotective (brain), cardioprotective (heart), gastroprotective (stomach), and musculoskeletal protective (joints, ligaments and muscles)

- Improves sleep

- Promotes a balanced inflammatory response

- Improves bone density

Research Side Effects

- Redness, itchiness, and swelling of injection sites

- Water retention

- Facial flushing

- Stimulates ghrelin

- Increases in stress responses through an increase in prolactin, ACTH and cortisol

- Sharp increase in IGF-1 levels

Matthew's Personal Insight on Research Dosing

- Tesamorelin

  - ¤ 500-2000 mcg per injection

- GHRP-6

  - ¤ 100 mcg per injection

- BPC-157

  - ¤ 300-600 mcg per injection

  - ¤ For an injury: Split dose into 200-300 mcg and inject around the area

Matthew's Personal Insight on Research Cycling

- Tesamorelin, GHRP-6

  - ¤ Multiple injections can be given a day to increase GH secretion. Often used in bodybuilding

- ¤ Carbohydrates and fatty acids can blunt growth hormone release. Best taken 30 minutes before eating and/or 2 hours after eating

  - ¤ 5 days on, 2 days off, 10-12 weeks on, 4-8 weeks off

- BPC-157

  - ¤ 5 days on, 2 days off, 10-12 weeks on, 4-8 weeks off

  - ¤ It can be cycled continuously

  - ¤ Best to take when the body needs recovery (post-workout, recovery days, before bed)

Matthew's Personal Insight on Research Timing & Benefits

- Burning Fat

  - ¤ Before a workout in a fasted state

- Building Muscle

  - ¤ After a workout in a fasted state

  - ¤ Best time to take BPC-157

- Sleep

  - ¤ Before bed in a fasted state

- General Anti-Aging

  - ¤ In the morning in a fasted state

Matthew's Opinion

- Tesamorelin is a nice upgrade replacement from MOD-GRF-1-29. I would start with a more conservative dosing scheme and increase as I felt more comfortable

- I like how GHRP-6 stimulates hunger with fewer side effects than GHRP-2

- I like how BPC-157 enhances the recovery aspect, leading to better gains and enhances growth hormone absorption

- I would switch out GHRP-6 with Ipamorelin throughout the week (3 days GHRP-6, 2 days Ipamorelin) to monitor bulk unless trying to do a massive bulk

Tesamorelin + GHRP-2 + BPC-157

Overview

- Tesamorelin is a GHRH (Growth Hormone Releasing Hormone)

- GHRP-2 is the second strongest GHRP (Growth Hormone Releasing Peptide)

- BPC-157 stands for body-protective compound. It was discovered in the human gastric juice

Why Add These Together?

- Tesamorelin goes up to the anterior pituitary gland and signals the body to create hormone (Stronger than MOD-GRF-1-29)

- GHRP-2 works by inhibiting somatostatin on the hypothalamus to allow the release of growth hormone

- GHRP-2 increases hunger and has a stronger release of growth hormone than GHRP-6 and Ipamorelin, making this a powerful combo for muscle-building

- BPC-157 enhances growth hormone absorption while adding neuroprotective (brain), cardioprotective (heart), gastroprotective (stomach), and musculoskeletal protective (joints, ligaments and muscles) benefits

- Combining these peptides ensures the creation and release of growth hormone occur simultaneously while adding enhanced growth hormone absorption and full body recovery

Research Benefits

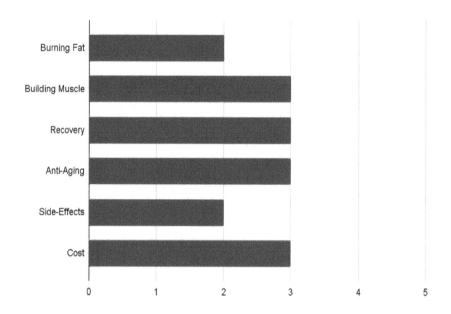

- Increase in the creation and release of endogenous growth hormone

- Promotes muscle growth

- Helps with mood and stress resilience

- Slows down aging

- Neuroprotective (brain), cardioprotective (heart), gastroprotective (stomach), and musculoskeletal protective (joints, ligaments and muscles)

- Improves sleep

- Promotes a balanced inflammatory response

- Improves bone density

Research Side Effects

- Itchiness and swelling of injection sites

- Water retention

- Facial flushing

- Stimulates ghrelin

- Increases in stress responses through an increase in prolactin, ACTH, and cortisol

- A sharp increase in IGF-1 levels

Matthew's Personal Insight on Research Dosing

- Tesamorelin

  - ¤ 500-2000 mcg per injection

- GHRP-2

  - ¤ 100 mcg per injection

- BPC-157

  - ¤ 300-600 mcg per injection

  - ¤ For an injury: Split the dose into 200-300 mcg and inject around the area

Matthew's Personal Insight on Research Cycling

- Tesamorelin, GHRP-6

  - ¤ Multiple injections can be given a day to increase GH secretion. Often used in bodybuilding

- Carbohydrates and fatty acids can blunt growth hormone release. Best taken 30 minutes before eating and/or 2 hours after eating

- 5 days on, 2 days off, 10-12 weeks on, 4-8 weeks off

- BPC-157

  - 5 days on, 2 days off, 10-12 weeks on, 4-8 weeks off

  - It can be cycled continuously

  - Best to take when the body needs recovery (post-workout, recovery days, before bed)

Matthew's Personal Insight on Research Timing & Benefits

- Burning Fat

  - Before a workout in a fasted state

- Building Muscle

  - After a workout in a fasted state

  - Best time to take BPC-157

- Sleep

  - Before bed in a fasted state

- General Anti-Aging

  - In the morning in a fasted state

Matthew's Opinion

- Tesamorelin is a nice upgrade replacement from MOD-GRF-1-29. I would start with a more conservative dosing scheme and increase as I felt more comfortable

- It is important to monitor closely when using GHRP-2, since prolonged use can lead to more side-effects.

- I would stick to shorter cycles when using GHRP-2, since it is a stronger GHRP and has more side effects compared to Ipamorelin

- I like how BPC-157 enhances the recovery aspect, leading to better gains and enhances growth hormone absorption

- I would switch out GHRP-2 with Ipamorelin throughout the week (3 days GHRP-2, 2 days Ipamorelin) to still get the stronger growth hormone release while reducing the unwanted side-effects that may happen from GHRP-2

Tesamorelin + Ipamorelin + BPC-157 + DSIP + Kisspeptin-10

Overview

- Tesamorelin is a GHRH (Growth Hormone Releasing Hormone)

- Ipamorelin is the mildest of GHRPs (Growth Hormone Releasing Peptide)

- BPC-157 stands for body-protective compound. It was discovered in the human gastric juice

- DSIP stands for Delta Sleep-Inducing Peptide

- Kisspeptin-10 is a neuropeptide hormone from the hypothalamus and is often called the "puberty" peptide

Why Add These Together?

- Tesamorelin goes up to the anterior pituitary gland and signals the body to create growth hormone (Stronger than MOD-GRF-1-29)

- Ipamorelin works by inhibiting somatostatin on the hypothalamus to allow the release of growth hormone

- Kisspeptin-10 stimulates the release of LH (Luteinizing Hormone) and FSH (Follicle Stimulating Hormone) in the pituitary, resulting in increased testosterone

- DSIP has been shown to increase endocrine functions during sleep, leading to higher releases of growth hormone, thyroid hormone, and testosterone. And DSIP helps aid in falling and staying asleep

- BPC-157 enhances growth hormone absorption while adding neuroprotective (brain), cardioprotective (heart), gastroprotective (stomach), and musculoskeletal protective (joints, ligaments and muscles) benefits

- Combining these peptides ensures the creation and release of growth hormone occur simultaneously, enhancing endogenous testosterone production while adding enhanced growth hormone absorption, full body recovery, and deeper sleep with larger releases of growth hormone and testosterone during sleep

Research Benefits

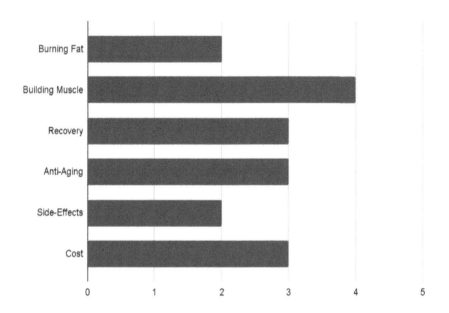

- Increase in the creation and release of endogenous growth hormone

- Promotes muscle growth

- Helps with mood and stress resilience

- Slows down aging

- Neuroprotective (brain), cardioprotective (heart), gastroprotective (stomach), and musculoskeletal protective (joints, ligaments and muscles)

- Improves sleep quality

- Improves bone density

- Stimulates LH (Luteinizing Hormone), FSH (Follicle Stimulating Hormone) and GHRH (Growth Hormone Releasing Hormone)

Research Side Effects

- Redness, itchiness, and swelling of injection sites

- Water retention

- Facial flushing

- May disrupt sleep

- Increases in stress responses through an increase in prolactin, ACTH, and cortisol

- A sharp increase in IGF-1 levels

Matthew's Personal Insight on Research Dosing

- Tesamorelin

  ¤ 500-2000 mcg per injection

- Ipamorelin

  ¤ 100-300 mcg per injection

- BPC-157

  ¤ 300-600 mcg per injection

- For an injury: Split the dose into 200-300 mcg and inject around the area

- DSIP
  - 100 mcg 3 hours before bed daily
  - Reduce down to 50 mcg 1x weekly once sleep stabilizes

- Kisspeptin-10
  - .1 mcg per kg

Matthew's Personal Insight on Research Cycling

- Tesamorelin, Ipamorelin
  - Multiple injections can be given a day to increase GH secretion. Often used in bodybuilding
  - Carbohydrates and fatty acids can blunt growth hormone release. Best taken 30 minutes before eating and/or 2 hours after eating
  - 5 days on, 2 days off, 10-12 weeks on, 4-8 weeks off

- BPC-157
  - 5 days on, 2 days off, 10-12 weeks on, 4-8 weeks off
  - It can be cycled continuously
  - Best to take when the body needs recovery (post-workout, recovery days, before bed)

- DSIP
  - Only used until sleep stabilizes
  - Reduce dose and frequency as sleep improves

- Kisspeptin-10

¤ Best taken in a fasted state in the morning to mimic natural testosterone production

¤ 3-5x week, 1 month on, 1 month off

Matthew's Personal Insight on Research Timing & Benefits

- Burning Fat

    ¤ Before a workout in a fasted state

- Building Muscle

    ¤ After a workout in a fasted state

    ¤ Best time to take BPC-157

- Sleep

    ¤ Before bed in a fasted state

    ¤ Only time to take DSIP - 3 hours before bed

- General Anti-Aging

    ¤ In the morning in a fasted state

Matthew's Opinion

- Tesamorelin is a nice upgrade replacement from MOD-GRF-1-29. I would start with a more conservative dosing scheme and increase as I felt more comfortable

- Ipamorelin is my favorite GHRP, as it allows for the release of growth hormone while being the safest GHRP

- DSIP is a great peptide to add to this muscle-building protocol. It is fairly inexpensive, deepens sleep, and enhances growth hormone and testosterone secretion

- I like how BPC-157 enhances the recovery aspect, leading to better gains while enhancing growth hormone absorption

- Kisspeptin-10 mechanism of action seems promising since it starts the testosterone cascade effect

- Overall, this is a peptide combo that I plan to use soon.

Tesamorelin + GHRP-6 + BPC-157 + DSIP + Kisspeptin-10 + PEG-MGF

Overview

- Tesamorelin is a GHRH (Growth Hormone Releasing Hormone)

- GHRP-6 is the third strongest GHRP (Growth Hormone Releasing Peptide)

- BPC-157 stands for body-protective compound. It was discovered in the human gastric juice

- DSIP stands for Delta Sleep-Inducing Peptide

- Kisspeptin-10 is a neuropeptide hormone from the hypothalamus and is often called the "puberty" peptide

- PEG-MGF is a split variant of IGF-1 (insulin-like growth factor) IGF-1 -> MGF

Why Add These Together?

- Tesamorelin goes up to the anterior pituitary gland and signals the body to create growth hormone (Stronger than MOD-GRF-1-29)

- GHRP-6 works by inhibiting somatostatin on the hypothalamus to allow the release of growth hormone

- GHRP-6 increases hunger, making this a great addition if bulking is the main focus

- Kisspeptin-10 stimulates the release of LH (Luteinizing Hormone) and FSH (Follicle Stimulating Hormone) in the pituitary, resulting in increased testosterone

- DSIP has been shown to increase endocrine functions during sleep, leading to higher releases of growth hormone, thyroid hormone, and testosterone. And DSIP helps aid in falling and staying asleep

- BPC-157 enhances growth hormone absorption while adding neuroprotective (brain), cardioprotective (heart), gastroprotective (stomach), and musculoskeletal protective (joints, ligaments and muscles) benefits

- PEG-MGF enhances muscle regeneration, activation, and proliferation of satellite stem cells. This results in faster muscle growth and repair

- Combining these peptides ensures the creation and release of growth hormone occur simultaneously, enhancing endogenous testosterone production and increasing muscle regeneration while enhancing growth hormone absorption, full body recovery, and deeper sleep with larger releases of growth hormone and testosterone during sleep

Research Benefits

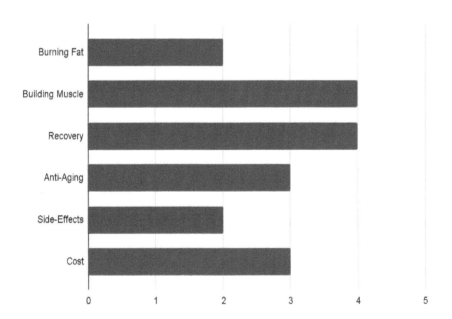

- Increase the creation and release of endogenous growth hormone

- Promotes muscle growth and repair

- Helps with mood and stress resilience

- Slows down aging

- Neuroprotective (brain), cardioprotective (heart), gastroprotective (stomach), and musculoskeletal protective (joints, ligaments and muscles)

- Improves sleep quality

- Improves bone density

- Stimulates LH (Luteinizing Hormone), FSH (Follicle Stimulating Hormone) and GHRH (Growth Hormone Releasing Hormone)

Research Side Effects

- Redness, itchiness, and swelling of injection sites

- Water retention

- Facial flushing

- May disrupt sleep

- Increases in stress responses through an increase in prolactin, ACTH, and cortisol

- A sharp increase in IGF-1 levels

Matthew's Personal Insight on Research Dosing

- Tesamorelin

    - 500-2000 mcg per injection

- GHRP-6

  - 100 mcg per injection

- BPC-157

  - 300-600 mcg per injection

  - For an injury: Split the dose into 200-300 mcg and inject around the area

- PEG-MGF

  - 100-600 mcg per injection

  - It can be split into separate 100 mcg injections to target different muscles

  - Suq-Q or IM muscle injections

- DSIP

  - 100 mcg 3 hours before bed daily

  - Reduce down to 50 mcg 1x weekly once sleep stabilizes

- Kisspeptin-10

  - .1 mcg per kg

Matthew's Personal Insight on Research Cycling

- Tesamorelin, GHRP-6

  - Multiple injections can be given a day to increase GH secretion. Often used in bodybuilding

  - Carbohydrates and fatty acids can blunt growth hormone release. Best taken 30 minutes before eating and/or 2 hours after eating

  - 5 days on, 2 days off, 10-12 weeks on, 4-8 weeks off

- BPC-157

  - 5 days on, 2 days off, 10-12 weeks on, 4-8 weeks off

  - It can be cycled continuously

  - Best to take when the body needs recovery (post-workout, recovery days, before bed)

- PEG-MGF

  - 2-3x week, 10-12 weeks on, 4-8 weeks off

  - Best taken post-workout or on recovery days

- DSIP

  - Only used until sleep stabilizes

  - Reduce dose and frequency as sleep improves

- Kisspeptin-10

  - Best taken in a fasted state in the morning to mimic natural testosterone production

  - 3-5x week, 1 month on, 1 month off

Matthew's Personal Insight on Research Timing & Benefits

- Burning Fat

  - Before a workout in a fasted state

- Building Muscle

  - After a workout in a fasted state

  - Best time to take BPC-157

- ⌷ Since PGF-MGF is a variant of IGF-1, I do not use pre-workout since IGF-1 and PGF-MGF will fight for the same receptors

- ⌷ Rest days are the best way to get the most out of PEG-MGF since IGF-1 will be lower

- Sleep

  - ⌷ Before bed in a fasted state

  - ⌷ Only time to take DSIP - 3 hours before bed

Matthew's Opinion

- Tesamorelin is a nice upgrade replacement from MOD-GRF-1-29. I would start with a more conservative dosing scheme and increase as I felt more comfortable

- I like how GHRP-6 stimulates hunger with fewer side effects than GHRP-2

- PEG-MGF is a great peptide to enhance muscle recovery and growth. I would use this on my recovery days

- DSIP is a great peptide to add to this muscle-building protocol. It is fairly inexpensive, deepens sleep, and enhances growth hormone and testosterone secretion

- I like how BPC-157 enhances the recovery aspect, leading to better gains while enhancing growth hormone absorption

- Kisspeptin-10 mechanism of action seems promising since it starts the testosterone cascade effect

- I would switch out GHRP-6 with Ipamorelin throughout the week (3 days GHRP-6, 2 days Ipamorelin) to monitor bulk unless trying to do a massive bulk

Tesamorelin + GHRP-2 + BPC-157 + DSIP + Kisspeptin-10 + PEG-MGF

Overview

- Tesamorelin is a GHRH (Growth Hormone Releasing Hormone)

- GHRP-2 is the second strongest GHRP (Growth Hormone Releasing Peptide)

- BPC-157 stands for body-protective compound. It was discovered in the human gastric juice

- DSIP stands for Delta Sleep-Inducing Peptide

- Kisspeptin-10 is a neuropeptide hormone from the hypothalamus and is often called the "puberty" peptide

- PEG-MGF is a split variant of IGF-1 (insulin-like growth factor) IGF-1 -> MGF

Why Add These Together?

- Tesamorelin goes up to the anterior pituitary gland and signals the body to create growth hormone (Stronger than MOD-GRF-1-29)

- GHRP-2 works by inhibiting somatostatin on the hypothalamus to allow the release of growth hormone

- GHRP-2 increases hunger and has a stronger release of growth hormone than GHRP-6 and Ipamorelin, making this a powerful combo for muscle-building

- Kisspeptin-10 stimulates the release of LH (Luteinizing Hormone) and FSH (Follicle Stimulating Hormone) in the pituitary, resulting in increased testosterone

- DSIP has been shown to increase endocrine functions during sleep, leading to higher releases of growth hormone, thyroid hormone, and testosterone. And DSIP helps aid in falling and staying asleep

- BPC-157 enhances growth hormone absorption while adding neuroprotective (brain), cardioprotective (heart), gastroprotective (stomach), and musculoskeletal protective (joints, ligaments and muscles) benefits

- PEG-MGF enhances muscle regeneration, activation, and proliferation of satellite stem cells. This results in faster muscle growth and repair

- Combining these peptides ensures the creation and release of growth hormone occur simultaneously, enhancing endogenous testosterone production and increasing muscle regeneration while enhancing growth hormone absorption, full body recovery, and deeper sleep with larger releases of growth hormone and testosterone during sleep

Research Benefits

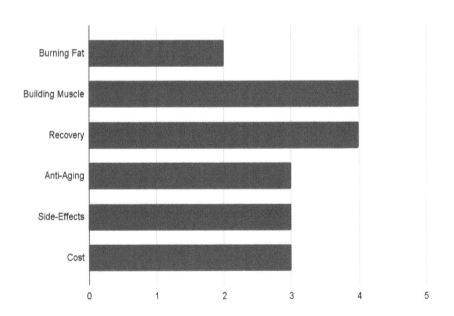

- Increase in the creation and release of endogenous growth hormone

- Promotes muscle growth and repair

- Helps with mood and stress resilience

- Slows down aging

- Neuroprotective (brain), cardioprotective (heart), gastroprotective (stomach), and musculoskeletal protective (joints, ligaments and muscles)

- Improves sleep quality

- Improves bone density

- Stimulates LH (Luteinizing Hormone), FSH (Follicle Stimulating Hormone) and GHRH (Growth Hormone Releasing Hormone)

Research Side Effects

- Redness, itchiness, and swelling of injection sites

- Water retention

- Facial flushing

- Stimulates hunger

- May disrupt sleep

- Increases in stress responses through an increase in prolactin, ACTH, and cortisol

- A sharp increase in IGF-1 levels

Matthew's Personal Insight on Research Dosing

- Tesamorelin

  - 500-2000 mcg per injection

- GHRP-2

  - 100 mcg per injection

- BPC-157

  - 300-600 mcg per injection

  - For an injury: Split the dose into 200-300 mcg and inject around the area

- PEG-MGF

  - 100-600 mcg per injection

  - It can be split into separate 100 mcg injections to target different muscles

  - Suq-Q or IM muscle injections

- DSIP

  - 100 mcg 3 hours before bed daily

  - Reduce down to 50 mcg 1x weekly once sleep stabilizes

- Kisspeptin-10

  - .1 mcg per kg (100-200 mcg for most people)

Matthew's Personal Insight on Research Cycling

- Tesamorelin, GHRP-2

  - Multiple injections can be given a day to increase GH secretion. Often used in bodybuilding

  - Carbohydrates and fatty acid can blunt growth hormone release. Best taken 30 minutes before eating and/or 2 hours after eating

  - 5 days on, 2 days off, 10-12 weeks on, 4-8 weeks off

- BPC-157

  - 5 days on, 2 days off, 10-12 weeks on, 4-8 weeks off

  - It can be cycled continuously

  - Best to take when body needs recovery (post-workout, recovery days, before bed)

- PEG-MGF

  - 2-3x week, 10-12 weeks on, 4-8 weeks off

  - Best taken post-workout or on recovery days

- DSIP

  - Only used until sleep stabilizes

  - Reduce dose and frequency as sleep improves

- Kisspeptin-10

  - Best taken in a fasted state in the morning to mimic natural testosterone production

Matthew's Personal Insight on Research Timing & Benefits

- Burning Fat

  - Before a workout in a fasted state

- Building Muscle

  - After a workout in a fasted state

  - Best time to take BPC-157

  - Since PGF-MGF is a variant of IGF-1, I do not want to use pre-workout since IGF-1 and PGF-MGF will fight for the same receptors.

  - Rest days are the best way to get the most out of PEG-MGF since IGF-1 will be lower

- Sleep

  - Before bed in a fasted state

  - Only time to take DSIP - 3 hours before bed

Matthew's Opinion

- Tesamorelin is a nice upgrade replacement from MOD-GRF-1-29. I would start with a more conservative dosing scheme and increase as I felt more comfortable

- It is important to monitor closely when using GHRP-2, since prolonged use can lead to more side-effects

- I would stick to shorter cycles when using GHRP-2, since it is a stronger GHRP and has more side effects compared to Ipamorelin & GHRP-6

- I would switch out GHRP-2 with Ipamorelin throughout the week (3 days GHRP-2, 2 days Ipamorelin) to still get the stronger growth hormone release while reducing the unwanted side-effects that may happen from GHRP-2

- PEG-MGF is a great peptide to enhance muscle recovery and growth. I would use this on my recovery days

- DSIP is a great peptide to add to this muscle-building protocol. It is fairly inexpensive, deepens sleep and enhances growth hormone and testosterone secretion

- I like how BPC-157 enhances the recovery aspect, leading to better gains while enhancing growth hormone absorption

- Kisspeptin-10 mechanism of action seems promising since it starts the testosterone cascade effect

Tesamorelin+ Ipamorelin + BPC-157 + DSIP + Kisspeptin-10 + PEG-MGF + IGF-LR3

Overview

- BPC-157 stands for body-protective compound. It was discovered in the human gastric juice

- Tesamorelin is a GHRH (Growth Hormone Releasing Hormone)

- Ipamorelin is the mildest of GHRPs (Growth Hormone Releasing Peptide)

- DSIP stands for Delta Sleep-Inducing Peptide

- Kisspeptin-10 is a neuropeptide hormone from the hypothalamus and is often called the "puberty" peptide

- PEG-MGF is a split variant of IGF-1 (insulin-like growth factor) IGF-1 -> MGF

- IGF-1 LR3 is a derivative of IGF-1 (released from the liver in response to growth hormone)

Why Add These Together?

- Tesamorelin goes up to the anterior pituitary gland and signals the body to create growth hormone (Stronger than MOD-GRF-1-29)

- Ipamorelin works by inhibiting somatostatin on the hypothalamus to allow the release of growth hormone

- Kisspeptin-10 stimulates the release of LH (Luteinizing Hormone) and FSH (Follicle Stimulating Hormone) in the pituitary, resulting in increased testosterone

- DSIP has been shown to increase endocrine functions during sleep, leading to higher releases of growth hormone, thyroid hormone, and testosterone. And DSIP helps aid in falling and staying asleep

- IGF-1 LR3 works by binding to IGF-1 receptors on muscle cells. This enhances protein synthesis and inhibits protein breakdown

- BPC-157 enhances growth hormone absorption while adding neuroprotective (brain), cardioprotective (heart), gastroprotective (stomach), and musculoskeletal protective (joints, ligaments and muscles) benefits

- PEG-MGF enhances muscle regeneration, activation and proliferation of satellite stem cells. This results in faster muscle growth and repair

- Combining these peptides ensures the creation and release of growth hormone occur simultaneously, enhances endogenous testosterone production, increases muscle regeneration, and prevents muscle breakdown while adding enhanced growth hormone absorption, full body recovery, deeper sleep with larger releases of growth hormone and testosterone during sleep

Research Benefits

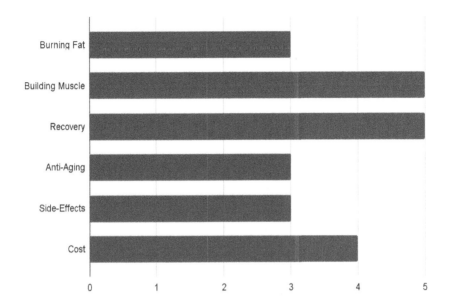

- Increase the creation and release of endogenous growth hormone

- Promotes muscle growth repair and prevents breakdown

- Helps with mood and stress resilience

- Slows down aging

- Neuroprotective (brain), cardioprotective (heart), gastroprotective (stomach), and musculoskeletal protective (joints, ligaments and muscles)

- Improves sleep quality

- Improves bone density

- Stimulates LH (Luteinizing Hormone), FSH (Follicle Stimulating Hormone) and GHRH (Growth Hormone Releasing Hormone)

Research Side Effects

- Redness, itchiness, and swelling of injection sites

- Water retention

- Facial flushing

- May disrupt sleep

- Increases in stress responses through an increase in prolactin, ACTH, and cortisol

- A sharp increase in IGF-1 levels

- Desensitization of GH receptors

Matthew's Personal Insight on Research Dosing

- Tesamorelin

  - 500-2000 mcg per injection

- Ipamorelin

  - 100-300 mcg per injection

- IGF-LR3

  - 20-60 mcg per injection

- BPC-157

  - 300-600 mcg per injection

  - For an injury: Split the dose into 200-300 mcg and inject around the area

- PEG-MGF

  - 100-600 mcg per injection

- It can be split into separate 100 mcg injections to target different muscles

- Suq-Q or IM muscle injections

- DSIP

  - 100 mcg 3 hours before bed daily

  - Reduce down to 50 mcg 1x weekly once sleep stabilizes

- Kisspeptin-10

  - .1 mcg per kg

Matthew's Personal Insight on Research Cycling

- Tesamorelin, Ipamorelin

  - Multiple injections can be given a day to increase GH secretion. Often used in bodybuilding

  - Carbohydrates and fatty acids can blunt growth hormone release. Best taken 30 minutes before eating or 2 hours after eating

  - 5 days on, 2 days off, 10-12 weeks on, 4-8 weeks off

- BPC-157

  - 5 days on, 2 days off, 10-12 weeks on, 4-8 weeks off

  - It can be cycled continuously

  - Best to take when the body needs recovery (post-workout, recovery days, before bed)

- IGF-LR3

  - 5 days on, 2 days off, 3-6 weeks on, 3-6 weeks off

  - Best taken with food after a workout for best results

- PEG-MGF

  - 2-3x week, 10-12 weeks on, 4-8 weeks off

  - Best taken post-workout or on recovery days

- DSIP

  - Only used until sleep stabilizes

  - Reduce dose and frequency as sleep improves

- Kisspeptin-10

  - Best taken in a fasted state in the morning to mimic natural testosterone production

  - 3-5x week, 1 month on, 1 month off

Matthew's Personal Insight on Research Timing & Benefits

- Burning Fat

  - Before a workout in a fasted state

- Building Muscle

  - After a workout in a fasted state (except for IGF-LR3)

  - Best time to take BPC-157

  - Since PGF-MGF is a variant of IGF-1, I do not want to use pre-workout since IGF-1 and PGF-MGF will fight for the same receptors

- ¤ Rest days are the best way to get the most out of PEG-MGF since IGF-1 will be lower

- Sleep

  - ¤ Before bed in a fasted state

Matthew's Opinion

- Tesamorelin is a nice upgrade replacement from MOD-GRF-1-29. I would start with a more conservative dosing scheme and increase as I felt more comfortable

- Ipamorelin is my favorite GHRP, as it allows for the release of growth hormone while being the safest GHRP

- PEG-MGF is a great peptide to enhance muscle recovery and growth. I would use this on my recovery days

- DSIP is a great peptide to add to this muscle-building protocol. It is fairly inexpensive, deepens sleep, and enhances growth hormone and testosterone secretion

- I like how BPC-157 enhances the recovery aspect, leading to better gains while enhancing growth hormone absorption

- Kisspeptin-10 mechanism of action seems promising since it starts the testosterone cascade effect

- I would use IGF-1 LR3 once more experience is gained with GH peptides and peptides in general. I would use this peptide 2-3x a week, focusing on the lower dose and cycle schemes

Tesamorelin + GHRP-6 + BPC-157 + DSIP + Kisspeptin-10 + PEG-MGF + IGF-LR3

Overview

- Tesamorelin is a GHRH (Growth Hormone Releasing Hormone)

- GHRP-6 is the third strongest GHRP (Growth Hormone Releasing Peptide)

- BPC-157 stands for body-protective compound. It was discovered in the human gastric juice

- DSIP stands for Delta Sleep-Inducing Peptide

- Kisspeptin-10 is a neuropeptide hormone from the hypothalamus and is often called the "puberty" peptide

- PEG-MGF is a split variant of IGF-1 (insulin-like growth factor) IGF-1 -> MGF

- IGF-1 LR3 is a derivative of IGF-1 (released from the liver in response to growth hormone)

Why Add These Together?

- Tesamorelin goes up to the anterior pituitary gland and signals the body to create growth hormone (Stronger than MOD-GRF-1-29)

- GHRP-6 works by inhibiting somatostatin on the hypothalamus to allow the release of growth hormone

- GHRP-6 increases hunger, making this a great addition if bulking is the main focus

- Kisspeptin-10 stimulates the release of LH (Luteinizing Hormone) and FSH (Follicle Stimulating Hormone) in the pituitary, resulting in increased testosterone

- DSIP has been shown to increase endocrine functions during sleep, leading to higher releases of growth hormone, thyroid hormone, and testosterone. And DSIP helps aid in falling and staying asleep

- IGF-1 LR3 works by binding to IGF-1 receptors on muscle cells This enhances protein synthesis and inhibits protein breakdown.

- BPC-157 enhances growth hormone absorption while adding neuroprotective (brain), cardioprotective (heart), gastroprotective (stomach), and musculoskeletal protective (joints, ligaments and muscles) benefits

- PEG-MGF enhances muscle regeneration, activation and proliferation of satellite stem cells. This results in faster muscle growth and repair

- Combining these peptides ensures the creation and release of growth hormone occur simultaneously, enhances endogenous testosterone production, increases muscle regeneration, and prevents muscle breakdown while enhancing growth hormone absorption, full body recovery, deeper sleep with larger releases of growth hormone and testosterone during sleep

Research Benefits

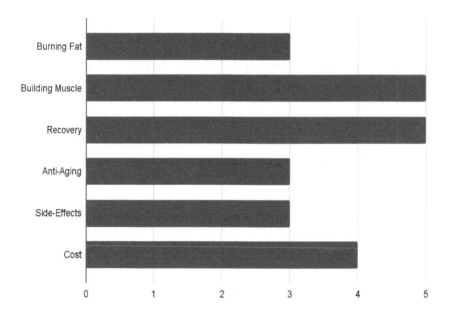

- Increase in the creation and release of endogenous growth hormone

- Promotes muscle growth repair and prevents breakdown

- Helps with mood and stress resilience

- Slows down aging

- Neuroprotective (brain), cardioprotective (heart), gastroprotective (stomach), and musculoskeletal protective (joints, ligaments and muscles)

- Improves sleep quality

- Improves bone density

- Stimulates LH (Luteinizing Hormone), FSH (Follicle Stimulating Hormone) and GHRH (Growth Hormone

Research Side Effects

- Redness, itchiness, and swelling of injection sites

- Water retention

- Facial flushing

- May disrupt sleep

- Increases hunger

- Increases in stress responses through an increase in prolactin, ACTH, and cortisol

- Sharp increase in IGF-1 levels

- Desensitization of GH receptors

Matthew's Personal Insight on Research Dosing

- Tesamorelin

    ¤ 500-2000 mcg per injection

- GHRP-6

    ¤ 100 mcg per injection

- IGF-LR3

    ¤ 20-60 mcg per injection

- BPC-157

    ¤ 300-600 mcg per injection

    ¤ For an injury: Split the dose into 200-300 mcg and inject around the area

- PEG-MGF

- ¤ 100-600 mcg per injection

- ¤ It can be split into separate 100 mcg injections to target different muscles

- ¤ Suq-Q or IM muscle injections

- DSIP

  - ¤ 100 mcg 3 hours before bed daily

  - ¤ Reduce down to 50 mcg 1x weekly once sleep stabilizes

- Kisspeptin-10

  - ¤ .1 mcg per kg (100-200 mcg for most people)

Matthew's Personal Insight on Research Cycling

- Tesamorelin, GHRP-6

  - ¤ Multiple injections can be given a day to increase GH secretion. Often used in bodybuilding

  - ¤ Carbohydrates and fatty acids can blunt growth hormone release. Best taken 30 minutes before eating or 2 hours after eating

  - ¤ 5 days on, 2 days off, 10-12 weeks on, 4-8 weeks off

- BPC-157

  - ¤ 5 days on, 2 days off, 10-12 weeks on, 4-8 weeks off

  - ¤ It can be cycled continuously

  - ¤ Best to take when the body needs recovery (post-workout, recovery days, before bed)

- IGF-LR3

  - ¤ 5 days on, 2 days off, 3-6 weeks on, 3-6 weeks off

- ¤ Best taken with food after a workout for best results

- PEG-MGF

  - ¤ 2-3x week, 10-12 weeks on, 4-8 weeks off

  - ¤ Best taken post-workout or on recovery days

- DSIP

  - ¤ Only used until sleep stabilizes

  - ¤ Reduce dose and frequency as sleep improves

- Kisspeptin-10

  - ¤ Best taken in a fasted state in the morning to mimic natural testosterone production

  - ¤ 3-5x week, 1 month on, 1 month off

Matthew's Personal Insight on Research Timing & Benefits

- Burning Fat

  - ¤ Before a workout in a fasted state

- Building Muscle

  - ¤ After a workout in a fasted state (except for IGF-LR3)

  - ¤ Best time to take BPC-157

  - ¤ Since PGF-MGF is a variant of IGF-1, I do not want to use pre-workout since IGF-1 and PGF-MGF will fight for the same receptors

  - ¤ Rest days are the best way to get the most out of PEG-MGF since IGF-1 will be lower

- Sleep

  ¤ Before bed in a fasted state

  ¤ Only time to take DSIP - 3 hours before bed

Matthew's Opinion

- Tesamorelin is a nice upgrade replacement from MOD-GRF-1-29. I would start with a more conservative dosing scheme and increase as I felt more comfortable

- I like how GHRP-6 stimulates hunger with fewer side-effects than GHRP-2

- I would switch out GHRP-6 with Ipamorelin throughout the week (3 days GHRP-6, 2 days Ipamorelin) to monitor bulk, unless trying to do a massive bulk

- PEG-MGF is a great peptide that enhances muscle recovery and growth. I would use this on my recovery days

- DSIP is a great peptide to add to this muscle-building protocol. It is fairly inexpensive, deepens sleep and enhances growth hormone and testosterone secretion

- I like how BPC-157 enhances the recovery aspect, leading to better gains while enhancing growth hormone absorption

- Kisspeptin-10 mechanism of action seems promising since it starts the testosterone cascade effect

- I would use IGF-1 LR3 once more experience is gained with GH peptides and peptides in general. I would use this peptide 2-3x a week, focusing on the lower dose and cycle schemes

Tesamorelin + GHRP-2 + BPC-157 + DSIP + Kisspeptin-10 + PEG-MGF + IGF-LR3

Overview

- Tesamorelin is a GHRH (Growth Hormone Releasing Hormone)

- GHRP-2 is the second strongest GHRP (Growth Hormone Releasing Peptide)

- BPC-157 stands for body-protective compound. It was discovered in the human gastric juice

- DSIP stands for Delta Sleep-Inducing Peptide

- Kisspeptin-10 is a neuropeptide hormone from the hypothalamus and is often called the "puberty" peptide

- PEG-MGF is a split variant of IGF-1 (insulin-like growth factor) IGF-1 -> MGF

- IGF-1 LR3 is a derivative of IGF-1 (released from the liver in response to growth hormone)

Why Add These Together?

- GHRP-2 works by inhibiting somatostatin on the hypothalamus to allow the release of growth hormone

- GHRP-2 increases hunger and has a stronger release of growth hormone than GHRP-6 and Ipamorelin, making this a powerful combo for muscle-building

- Tesamorelin goes up to the anterior pituitary gland and signals the body to create growth hormone (Stronger than MOD-GRF-1-29)

- Kisspeptin-10 stimulates the release of LH (Luteinizing Hormone) and FSH (Follicle Stimulating Hormone) in the pituitary, resulting in increased testosterone

- DSIP has been shown to increase endocrine functions during sleep, leading to higher releases of growth hormone, thyroid hormone, and testosterone. And DSIP helps aid in falling and staying asleep

- IGF-1 LR3 works by binding to IGF-1 receptors on muscle cells. This enhances protein synthesis and inhibits protein breakdown

- BPC-157 enhances growth hormone absorption while adding neuroprotective (brain), cardioprotective (heart), gastroprotective (stomach), and musculoskeletal protective (joints, ligaments and muscles) benefits

- PEG-MGF enhances muscle regeneration, activation and proliferation of satellite stem cells. This results in faster muscle growth and repair

- Combining these peptides ensures the creation and release of growth hormone occur simultaneously, enhancing endogenous testosterone production, increasing muscle regeneration, and preventing muscle breakdown while enhancing growth hormone absorption, full body recovery, deeper sleep with larger releases of growth hormone and testosterone during sleep

Research Benefits

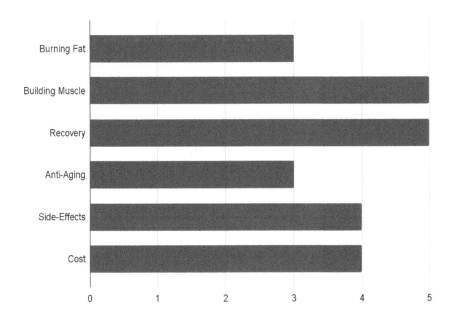

- Increase the creation and release of endogenous growth hormone

- Promotes muscle growth repair and prevents breakdown

- Helps with mood and stress resilience

- Slows down aging

- Neuroprotective (brain), cardioprotective (heart), gastroprotective (stomach), and musculoskeletal protective (joints, ligaments and muscles)

- Improves sleep quality

- Improves bone density

- Stimulates LH (Luteinizing Hormone), FSH (Follicle Stimulating Hormone) and GHRH (Growth Hormone Releasing Hormone)

Research Side Effects

- Redness, itchiness, and swelling of injection sites

- Water retention

- Facial flushing

- May disrupt sleep

- Increases hunger

- Increases in stress responses through an increase in prolactin, ACTH, and cortisol

- A sharp increase in IGF-1 levels

- Desensitization of GH receptors

- Prolonged use and over-saturation of receptors may increase anxiety and depression.

Matthew's Personal Insight on Research Dosing

- Tesamorelin

  ¤   500-2000 mcg per injection

- GHRP-2

  ¤   100 mcg per injection

- IGF-LR3

  ¤   20-60 mcg per injection

- BPC-157

  ¤   300-600 mcg per injection

- For an injury: Split the dose into 200-300 mcg and inject around the area

- PEG-MGF

  - 100-600 mcg per injection

  - It can be split into separate 100 mcg injections to target different muscles

  - Suq-Q or IM muscle injections

- DSIP

  - 100 mcg 3 hours before bed daily

  - Reduce down to 50 mcg 1x weekly once sleep stabilizes

- Kisspeptin-10

  - .1 mcg per kg

Matthew's Personal Insight on Research Cycling

- Tesamorelin, GHRP-2

  - Multiple injections can be given a day to increase GH secretion. Often used in bodybuilding

  - Carbohydrates and fatty acids can blunt growth hormone release. Best taken 30 minutes before eating or 2 hours after eating

  - 5 days on, 2 days off, 10-12 weeks on, 4-8 weeks off

- BPC-157

  - 5 days on, 2 days off, 10-12 weeks on, 4-8 weeks off

  - It can be cycled continuously

- ⌷ Best to take when the body needs recovery (post-workout, recovery days, before bed)

- IGF-LR3

  - ⌷ 5 days on, 2 days off, 3-6 weeks on, 3-6 weeks off

  - ⌷ Best taken with food after a workout for best results

- PEG-MGF

  - ⌷ 2-3x week, 10-12 weeks on, 4-8 weeks off

  - ⌷ Best taken post-workout or on recovery days

- DSIP

  - ⌷ Only used until sleep stabilizes

  - ⌷ Reduce dose and frequency as sleep improves

- Kisspeptin-10

  - ⌷ Best taken in a fasted state in the morning to mimic natural testosterone production

  - ⌷ 3-5x week, 1 month on, 1 month off

Matthew's Personal Insight on Research Timing & Benefits

- Burning Fat

  - ⌷ Before a workout in a fasted state

- Building Muscle

  - ⌷ After a workout in a fasted state (except for IGF-LR3)

  - ⌷ Best time to take BPC-157

- ¤ Since PGF-MGF is a variant of IGF-1, I do not want to use pre-workout since IGF-1 and PGF-MGF will fight for the same receptors.

- ¤ Rest days are the best way to get the most out of PEG-MGF since IGF-1 will be lower

- Sleep

- ¤ Before bed in a fasted state

- ¤ Only time to take DSIP - 3 hours before bed

Matthew's Opinion

- Tesamorelin is a nice upgrade replacement from MOD-GRF-1-29. I would start with a more conservative dosing scheme and increase as I got more comfortable

- It is important to monitor closely when using GHRP-2, since prolonged use can lead to more side-effects

- I would stick to shorter cycles when using GHRP-2, since it is a stronger GHRP and has more side effects compared to Ipamorelin and GHRP-6

- I would switch out GHRP-2 with Ipamorelin throughout the week (3 days GHRP-2, 2 days Ipamorelin) to still get the stronger growth hormone release while reducing the unwanted side-effects that may happen from GHRP-2

- PEG-MGF is a great peptide to enhance muscle recovery and growth. I would use this on my recovery days

- DSIP is a great peptide to add to this muscle-building protocol. It is fairly inexpensive, deepens sleep, and enhances growth hormone and testosterone secretion

- I like how BPC-157 enhances the recovery aspect, leading to better gains while enhancing growth hormone absorption

- Kisspeptin-10 mechanism of action seems promising since it starts the testosterone cascade effect

- I would use IGF-1 LR3 once more experience is gained with GH peptides and peptides in general. I would use this peptide 2-3x a week, focusing on the lower dose and cycle schemes

12. Peptides Combos for Longevity

Epithalon + BPC-157

Overview

- Epithalon is a synthetic peptide that reproduces the effects of epithalamion, a peptide found naturally in the pineal gland

- BPC-157 stands for body-protective compound. It was discovered in the human gastric juice

Why Add These Together?

- BPC-157 is neuroprotective (brain), cardioprotective (heart), gastroprotective (stomach), and musculoskeletal protective (joints, ligaments, and muscles)

- Epithalon increases the production of the enzyme telomerase, which helps cells to reproduce telomeres, resulting in increased longevity due to healthier telomeres since telomere length is correlated to increased lifespan

- Combining these peptides packs a powerful anti-aging benefit due to the increase in telomeres with additional full-body rejuvenation

Research Benefits

Benefits

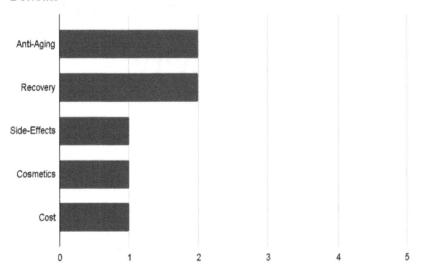

- Neuroprotective (brain), cardioprotective (heart), gastroprotective (stomach), and musculoskeletal protective (joints, ligaments and muscles)

- Decelerates aging

- Increase telomerase activity and elongation

- Normalizes melatonin levels

- Improve insulin sensitivity

- Prevents and treats cancer

- Promotes quality sleep

Research Side Effects

- Redness, itchiness, and swelling of the injection site

- Difficulty sleeping

- Fatigue

- Headache

- Water retention

Matthew's Personal Insight on Research Cycling & Dosing

- BPC-157

    - 400-600 mcg per injection

    - Take BPC-157 with 10-20 Epithalon cycle

- Epithalon

    - 50-100 mg total

    - 5-10 mg daily for 10-20 days

    - Recommended 1-2x a year to maximize longevity benefits

Matthew's Opinion

- This is an all-around great peptide stack for beginners who are looking into longevity

- Since Epithalon is designed to be taken in a 10–20-day cycle, I believe adding other healing peptides will enhance the overall protocol, making this a great protocol to run 1-2x a time year when I feel like I need a "tune-up"

- I would use Epithalon in a cycle of 20 days to get more doses of BPC-157.

Epithalon + BPC-157 + TB-500

Overview

- Epithalon is a synthetic peptide that reproduces the effects of epithalamion, a peptide found naturally in the pineal gland

- BPC-157 stands for body-protective compound. It was discovered in the human gastric juice

- Thymosin Beta-4 (TB-4) is related to thymosin, a hormone that is secreted by your thymus, with its primary function to produce T cells, which is an essential aspect of the immune system

Why Add These Together?

- BPC-157 is neuroprotective (brain), cardioprotective (heart), gastroprotective (stomach), and musculoskeletal protective (joints, ligaments and muscles)

- Epithalon increases the production of the enzyme telomerase, which helps cells to reproduce telomeres, resulting in increased longevity due to healthier telomeres since telomere length is correlated to increased lifespan

- Thymosin Beta-4 works by binding to actin, which is a protein that influences the action and formation of most cells in the body. Enhancing the mechanism of actin leads to faster healing time, especially in injured areas.

- Combining these peptides packs a powerful anti-aging benefit due to the increase in telomeres with additional full-body rejuvenation

Research Benefits

Benefits

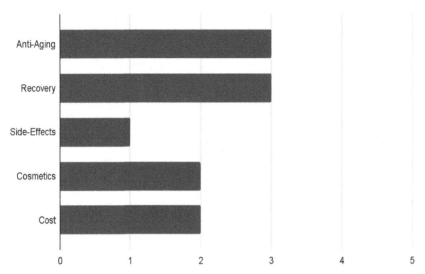

- Neuroprotective (brain), cardioprotective (heart), gastroprotective (stomach), and musculoskeletal protective (joints, ligaments and muscles)

- Decelerates aging

- Increase telomerase activity and elongation

- Normalizes melatonin levels

- Boosts the immune system

- Improves liver health

- Accelerates wound healing

- Improves eye health

- Promotes hair growth

Research Side Effects

- Redness, itchiness, and swelling of injection site

- Difficulty sleeping

- Fatigue

- Headache

- Water retention

- Temporary tiredness

Matthew's Personal Insight on Research Dosing & Cycling

- TB-4

  - 300 mcg to 1-gram subcutaneous injection

  - Take TB-4 with 10-20 day Epithalon cycle

- BPC-157

  - 400-600 mcg per subcutaneous injection

  - Take BPC-157 with 10-20 day Epithalon cycle

- Epithalon

  - 50-100 mg total

  - 5-10 mg daily for 10-20 days

  - Recommended to run 1-2x a year to maximize longevity benefits

Matthew's Opinion

- BPC-157 and TB-4 have a synergistic effect and are a powerful combo when it comes to healing and anti-aging

- Since Epithalon is designed to be taken in a 10–20-day cycle, adding other healing peptides will enhance the overall protocol, making this a great protocol to run 1-2x when I feel like I need a "tune-up."

- I would use Epithalon in a cycle of 20 days to get more doses of BPC-157 & TB-4.

Epithalon + BPC-157 + TB-500 + MOD-GRF + Ipamorelin

Overview

- Epithalon is a synthetic peptide that reproduces the effects of epithalamion, a peptide found naturally in the pineal gland

- BPC-157 stands for body-protective compound. It was discovered in the human gastric juice

- Thymosin Beta-4 (TB-4) is related to thymosin, a hormone secreted by your thymus, with its main function to produce T cells, which is an essential aspect of the immune system.

- MOD-GRF-1-29 is a GHRH (Growth Hormone Releasing Hormone)

- Ipamorelin is the mildest of GHRPs (Growth Hormone Releasing Peptide)

Why Add These Together?

- BPC-157 is neuroprotective (brain), cardioprotective (heart), gastroprotective (stomach), and musculoskeletal protective (joints, ligaments and muscles)

- Epithalon increases the production of the enzyme telomerase, which helps cells to reproduce telomeres, resulting in increased longevity due to healthier telomeres since telomere length is correlated to increased lifespan.

- Thymosin Beta-4 works by binding to actin, which is a protein that influences the action and formation of most cells in the body. Enhancing the mechanism of actin leads to faster healing time, especially in injured areas.

- MOD-GRF-1-29 goes up to the anterior pituitary gland and signals the body to create growth hormone

- Ipamorelin works by inhibiting somatostatin on the hypothalamus to allow the release of growth hormone

- Combining these peptides ensures the creation and release of growth hormone occur simultaneously, packs a powerful anti-aging benefit due to the increase in telomeres with additional full-body rejuvenation

Research Benefits

Benefits

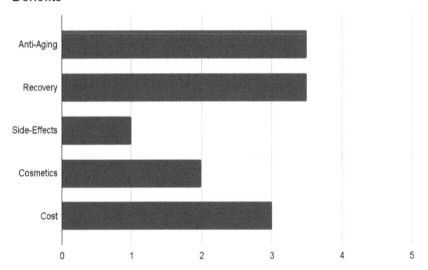

- Neuroprotective (brain), cardioprotective (heart), gastroprotective (stomach), and musculoskeletal protective (joints, ligaments and muscles)

- Decelerates aging

- Increase telomerase activity and elongation

- Normalizes melatonin levels

- Boosts the immune system

- Increase in the creation and release of endogenous growth hormone

- Accelerates wound healing

- Promotes muscle growth

- Promotes hair growth

Research Side Effects

- Redness, itchiness, and swelling of injection site

- Difficulty sleeping

- Fatigue

- Headache

- Water retention

- Temporary tiredness

Matthew's Personal Insight on Research Dosing

- MOD-GRF-1-29

  - 100 mcg per injection (more is not better)

- Ipamorelin

  - 100-300 mcg per injection

- TB-4

  - 300 mcg to 1-gram subcutaneous injection

- BPC-157

  - 400-600 mcg per subcutaneous injection

- Epithalon

  ¤ 50-100 mg total

  ¤ 5-10 mg daily for 10-20 days

Matthew's Personal Insight on Research Cycling

- Epithalon

  ¤ 10–20-day cycle

  ¤ Recommended to run 1-2x to maximize longetivity benefits

- TB-4, BPC-157, Ipamorelin, MOD-GRF-1-29

  ¤ Take daily with Epithalon cycle

- Ipamorelin, MOD-GRF-1-29

  ¤ Carbohydrates and fatty acids can blunt growth hormone release. Best taken 30 minutes before eating or 2 hours after eating

Matthew's Opinion

- Ipamorelin and MOD-GRF-1-29 are one of my favorite peptide combos for increasing endogenous growth hormone that I have used for several years on and off. It makes a great addition to add to this longevity stack

- BPC-157 and TB-4 have a synergistic effect and are a powerful combo when it comes to healing and anti-aging

- Since Epithalon is designed to be taken in a 10–20-day cycle, adding other healing peptides will enhance the overall protocol, making this a great protocol to run 1-2x when I feel like I need a "tune-up."

- I would use Epithalon in a cycle of 20 days to get more doses of the other peptides in the stack.

Epithalon + BPC-157 + TB-500 + Tesamorelin + Ipamorelin

Overview

- Epithalon is a synthetic peptide that reproduces the effects of epithalamion, a peptide found naturally in the pineal gland

- BPC-157 stands for body-protective compound. It was discovered in the human gastric juice

- Thymosin Beta-4 (TB-4) is related to thymosin, a hormone that is secreted by your thymus, with its main function to produce T cells, which is an essential aspect of the immune system

- Tesamorelin is a GHRH (Growth Hormone Releasing Hormone)

- Ipamorelin is the mildest of GHRP's (Growth Hormone Releasing Peptide)

Why Add These Together?

- BPC-157 is neuroprotective (brain), cardioprotective (heart), gastroprotective (stomach), and musculoskeletal protective (joints, ligaments and muscles)

- Epithalon increases the production of the enzyme telomerase, which helps cells to reproduce telomeres, resulting in increased longevity due to healthier telomeres since telomere length is correlated to increased lifespan

- Thymosin Beta-4 works by binding to actin, which is a protein that influences the action and formation of most cells in the body. Enhancing the mechanism of actin leads to faster healing time, especially in injured areas.

- Tesamorelin goes up to the anterior pituitary gland and signals the body to create growth hormone (Stronger than MOD-GRF-1-29)

- Ipamorelin works by inhibiting somatostatin on the hypothalamus to allow the release of growth hormone

- Combining these peptides ensures the creation and release of growth hormone occur simultaneously and packs a powerful anti-aging benefit due to the increase in telomeres with additional full-body rejuvenation

Research Benefits

Benefits

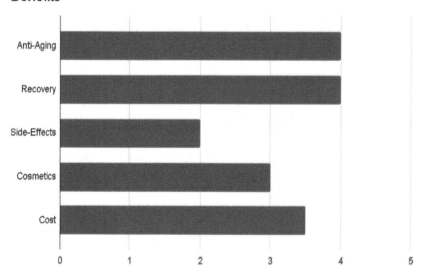

- Neuroprotective (brain), cardioprotective (heart), gastroprotective (stomach), and musculoskeletal protective (joints, ligaments and muscles)

- Decelerates aging

- Increase telomerase activity and elongation

- Normalizes melatonin levels

- Boosts the immune system

- Increase in the creation and release of endogenous growth hormone

- Accelerates wound healing

- Promotes muscle growth

- Promotes hair growth

Research Side Effects

- Redness, itchiness, and swelling of the injection site

- Difficulty sleeping

- Fatigue

- Headache

- Water retention

- Temporary tiredness

- A sharp increase in IGF-1 levels

Matthew's Personal Insight on Research Dosing

- Tesamorelin

  - 500-2000 mcg per subcutaneous injection

- Ipamorelin

  - 100-300 mcg per subcutaneous injection

- TB-4

  - 300 mcg to 1-gram subcutaneous injection

- BPC-157

  - ¤ 400-600 mcg per subcutaneous injection

- Epithalon

  - ¤ 50-100 mg total

  - ¤ 5-10 mg daily for 10-20 days

Matthew's Personal Insight on Research Cycling

- Epithalon

  - ¤ 10–20-day cycle

  - ¤ Recommended to run 1-2x a year to maximize longevity benefits

- TB-4, BPC-157, Ipamorelin, Tesamorelin

  - ¤ Take daily with Epithalon cycle

- Ipamorelin, Tesamorelin

  - ¤ Carbohydrates and fatty acids can blunt growth hormone release. Best taken 30 minutes before eating or 2 hours after eating

Matthew's Opinion

- Ipamorelin and Tesamorelin is the gold standard peptide combo for increasing endogenous growth hormone. It makes a great addition to add to this longevity stack

- Tesamorelin is a nice upgrade replacement from MOD-GRF-1-29. I would start with a more conservative dosing scheme and increase as I gained confidence

- BPC-157 and TB-4 have a synergistic effect and are a powerful combo when it comes to healing and anti-aging

- Since Epithalon is designed to be taken in a 10–20-day cycle, adding other healing peptides will enhance the overall protocol, making this a great protocol to run 1-2x when I feel like I need a "tune-up."

- I would use Epithalon in a cycle of 20 days so that I could get more doses of the other peptides in the stack

Epithalon + BPC-157 + TB-500 + Tesamorelin + Ipamorelin + GHK-CU

Overview

- Epithalon is a synthetic peptide that reproduces the effects of epithalamion, a peptide found naturally in the pineal gland

- BPC-157 stands for body-protective compound. It was discovered in the human gastric juice

- Thymosin Beta-4 (TB-4) is related to thymosin, a hormone that is secreted by your thymus, with its primary function to produce T cells, which is an essential aspect of the immune system

- Tesamorelin is a GHRH (Growth Hormone Releasing Hormone)

- Ipamorelin is the mildest of GHRPs (Growth Hormone Releasing Peptide)

- GHK-Cu is a naturally occurring copper peptide found in human plasma. As people age, they naturally lose the ability to produce this

Why Add These Together?

- BPC-157 is neuroprotective (brain), cardioprotective (heart), gastroprotective (stomach), and musculoskeletal protective (joints, ligaments and muscles)

- Epithalon increases the production of the enzyme telomerase, which helps cells to reproduce telomeres, resulting in increased longevity due to healthier telomeres since telomere length is correlated to increased lifespan

- Thymosin Beta-4 works by binding to actin, a protein that influences the action and formation of most cells in the body. Enhancing the mechanism of actin leads to faster healing time, especially in injured areas.

- GHK-Cu increases collagen, stem cell production, and bone formation by stimulating chondrocytes in bones. GHK-Cu blocks the release of oxidative damage and enhances angiogenesis (development of new blood cells)

- Tesamorelin goes up to the anterior pituitary gland and signals the body to create growth hormone (Stronger than MOD-GRF-1-29)

- Ipamorelin works by inhibiting somatostatin on the hypothalamus to allow the release of growth hormone

- Combining these peptides ensures the creation and release of growth hormone occur simultaneously, packs a powerful anti-aging benefit due to the increase in telomeres with additional full-body rejuvenation

Research Benefits

Benefits

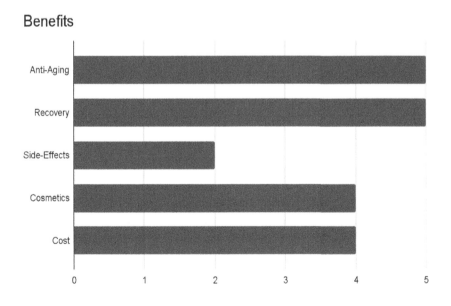

- Neuroprotective (brain), cardioprotective (heart), gastroprotective (stomach), and musculoskeletal protective (joints, ligaments and muscles)

- Tightens loose skin and enhances skin elasticity

- Increase telomerase activity and elongation

- Normalizes melatonin levels

- Boosts the immune system

- Increase the creation and release of endogenous growth hormone

- Accelerates wound healing

- Promotes muscle growth

- Promotes hair growth

Research Side Effects

- Redness, itchiness, and swelling of the injection site

- Difficulty sleeping

- Fatigue

- Headache

- Water retention

- Temporary tiredness

- A sharp increase in IGF-1 levels

- Possibility for copper toxicity

Matthew's Personal Insight on Research Dosing

- GHK-Cu

  - ¤ 1-2 mg per subcutaneous injection

- Tesamorelin

  - ¤ 500-2000 mcg per subcutaneous injection

- Ipamorelin

  - ¤ 100-300 mcg per subcutaneous injection

- TB-4

  - ¤ 300 mcg to 1-gram subcutaneous injection

- BPC-157

  - ¤ 400-600 mcg per subcutaneous injection

- Epithalon

  - ¤ 50-100 mg total

  - ¤ 5-10 mg daily for 10-20 days

Matthew's Personal Insight on Research Cycling

- Epithalon

  - ¤ 10–20-day cycle

  - ¤ Recommended to run 1-2x year to maximize longevity benefits

- TB-4, BPC-157, Ipamorelin, Tesamorelin, GHK-Cu

  - ¤ Take daily with Epithalon cycle

- Ipamorelin, Tesamorelin

  - ¤ Carbohydrates and fatty acids can blunt growth hormone release. Best taken 30 minutes before eating or 2 hours after eating

Matthew's Opinion

- Ipamorelin and Tesamorelin are the gold standard peptide combo for increasing endogenous growth hormone. It makes a great addition to add to this longevity stack

- Tesamorelin is a nice upgrade replacement from MOD-GRF-1-29. I would start with a more conservative dosing scheme and increase as I felt more comfortable.

- BPC-157 and TB-4 have a synergistic effect and are a powerful combo when it comes to healing and anti-aging

- GHK-Cu enhances the anti-aging, recovery, and cosmetic benefits of this stack. And I like how GHK-Cu can be applied topically and through an injection. I would use both forms when using this peptide combo if money was not a barrier

- Since Epithalon is designed to be taken in a 10–20-day cycle, adding other healing peptides will enhance the overall protocol, making this a great protocol to run 1-2x when I feel like I need a "tune-up.""

- I would use Epithalon in a cycle of 20 days to get more doses of the other peptides in the stack

Epithalon + BPC-157 + TB-500 + Tesamorelin + Ipamorelin + GHK-CU + Humanin

Overview

- Epithalon is a synthetic peptide that reproduces the effects of epithalamion, a peptide found naturally in the pineal gland

- BPC-157 stands for body-protective compound. It was discovered in the human gastric juice

- Thymosin Beta-4 (TB-4) is related to thymosin, a hormone that is secreted by your thymus, with its main function to produce T cells, which is an essential aspect of the immune system

- Tesamorelin is a GHRH (Growth Hormone Releasing Hormone)

- Ipamorelin is the mildest of GHRP's (Growth Hormone Releasing Peptide)

- GHK-Cu is a naturally occurring copper peptide found in human plasma. As people age, they naturally lose the ability to produce this

- Humanin is a peptide found naturally in the mitochondria and many other parts of the human body, such as the heart, kidney, brain, and skeletal muscles.

Why Add These Together?

- BPC-157 is neuroprotective (brain), cardioprotective (heart), gastroprotective (stomach), and musculoskeletal protective (joints, ligaments and muscles)

- Epithalon increases the production of the enzyme telomerase, which helps cells to reproduce telomeres, resulting in increased longevity due to healthier telomeres since telomere length is correlated to increased lifespan

- Thymosin Beta-4 works by binding to actin, which is a protein that influences the action and formation of most cells in the body. Enhancing the mechanism of actin leads to faster healing time, especially in injured areas.

- Humanin plays a role in returning the body to optimal function during a metabolic stress response and has been linked to largely influencing the health span and lifespan

- GHK-Cu increases collagen, stem cell production, and bone formation by stimulating chondrocytes in bones. GHK-Cu blocks the release of oxidative damage and enhances angiogenesis (development of new blood cells)

- Tesamorelin goes up to the anterior pituitary gland and signals the body to create growth hormone (Stronger than MOD-GRF-1-29)

- Ipamorelin works by inhibiting somatostatin on the hypothalamus to allow the release of growth hormone

- Combining these peptides ensures the creation and release of growth hormone occurs simultaneously and packs a powerful anti-aging benefit due to the increase in telomeres and restoration of mitochondrial damage with additional full-body rejuvenation

Research Benefits

Benefits

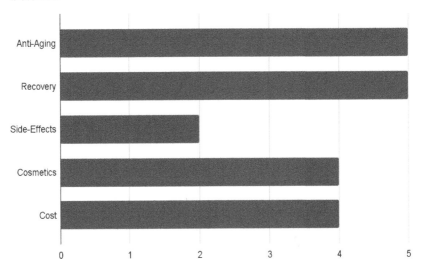

- Neuroprotective (brain), cardioprotective (heart), gastroprotective (stomach), and musculoskeletal protective (joints, ligaments and muscles)

- Tightens loose skin and enhances skin elasticity

- Increase telomerase activity and elongation

- Normalizes melatonin levels

- Boosts the immune system

- Increase in the creation and release of endogenous growth hormone

- Accelerates wound healing

- Promotes muscle growth

- Promotes hair growth

Research Side Effects

- Redness, itchiness, and swelling of the injection site

- Difficulty sleeping

- Fatigue

- Headache

- Water retention

- Temporary tiredness

- A sharp increase in IGF-1 levels

- Possibility for copper toxicity

Matthew's Personal Insight on Research Dosing

- GHK-Cu

  - 1-2 mg per subcutaneous injection

- Tesamorelin

  - 500-2000 mcg per subcutaneous injection

- Ipamorelin

  - 100-300 mcg per subcutaneous injection

- Humanin

  - .04 mg/kg as the therapeutic dose

  - Weigh 80kg -> 3.2 mg

  - Weigh 90 kg -> 3.6 mg

  - Weigh 100 kg -> 4 mg

- TB-4

  - ¤ 300 mcg to 1-gram subcutaneous injection

- BPC-157

  - ¤ 400-600 mcg per subcutaneous injection

- Epithalon

  - ¤ 50-100 mg total

  - ¤ 5-10 mg daily for 10-20 day

Matthew's Personal Insight on Research Cycling

- Epithalon

  - ¤ 10–20-day cycle

  - ¤ Recommended to run 1-2x a year to maximize longevity benefits

- TB-4, BPC-157, Ipamorelin, Tesamorelin, GHK-Cu, Humanin

  - ¤ Take daily with Epithalon cycle

- Ipamorelin, Tesamorelin

  - ¤ Carbohydrates and fatty acids can blunt growth hormone release. Best taken 30 minutes before eating or 2 hours after eating

Matthew's Opinion

- Ipamorelin and Tesamorelin are the gold standard peptide combo for increasing endogenous growth hormone. It makes a great addition to add to this longevity stack

- Tesamorelin is a nice upgrade replacement from MOD-GRF-1-29. I would start with a conservative dosing scheme and increase as I felt more comfortable

- BPC-157 and TB-4 have a synergistic effect and are a powerful combo when it comes to healing and anti-aging

- I like how Humanin has been linked to largely influencing the health span and lifespan. And it regulates and enhances mitochondrial health.

- GHK-Cu enhances the anti-aging, recovery, and cosmetic benefits of this stack. And I like how GHK-Cu can be applied topically and through an injection. I would use both forms when using this peptide combo if money was not a barrier

- Since Epithalon is designed to be taken in a 10–20-day cycle, adding other healing peptides will enhance the overall protocol, making this a great protocol to run 1-2x when I feel like I need a "tune-up."

- I would use Epithalon in a cycle of 20 days to get more doses of the other peptides in the stack

13. Peptides Combos for Brain Function

N-Acetyl Selank + BPC-157

Overview

- Selank was created from Tuftsin (a peptide that naturally comes from the antibody immunoglobulin G) with additional sequins to enhance the peptides' stability

- N-Acetyl Selank (added amide group) is better absorbed, more potent, and has a longer half-life than Selank

- BPC-157 stands for body-protective compound. It was discovered in the human gastric juice

Why Add These Together?

- Selank works by regulating neurotransmitter levels in the brain, including serotonin, dopamine, and GABA. Additionally, Selank enhances BDNF while reducing pain, inflammation, and cancerous development

- BPC-157 is neuroprotective (brain), cardioprotective (heart), gastroprotective (stomach), and musculoskeletal protective (joints, ligaments and muscles).

- BPC-157 is often used to treat TBIs and concussions

- Combining these peptides enhances learning, memory, and mood with additional full-body healing and protective benefits, especially regarding the brain

Research Benefits

Benefits

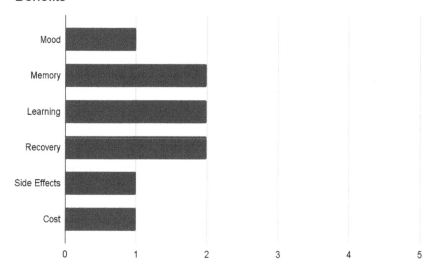

- Neuroprotective (brain), cardioprotective (heart), gastroprotective (stomach), and musculoskeletal protective (joints, ligaments and muscles)

- Increases BDNF

- Increases dopamine and serotonin signaling

- It can be used to help treat generalized anxiety disorder

- Enhanced learning and memory capacity

- Promotes healthy relaxation by increasing GABA

- Helps balance sleep vs. wakefulness

- Helps regulate inflammation and has anti-viral properties

Research Side Effects

- Redness, itchiness, and swelling of injection sites

- Water retention

- Excess and prolonged use of Selank can lead to desensitization.

Matthew's Personal Insight on Dosing & Cycling

- N-Acetyl Selank

  - 100-300 mcg through a subcutaneous injection

  - 750-1000 mcg through an intranasal spray (preferred method)

  - 6 weeks on, 6 weeks off

- BPC-157

  - 400-600 mcg per injection

  - Intended to take a 6-week cycle of Selank

- Best to take this peptide combo in the morning to prevent sleep disturbances

- Both can be taken through an intranasal spray

Matthew's Opinion

- This is a great beginner combo to focus on brain health

- I like how both of these peptides can be taken through an intranasal spray or injecting

- N-Acetyl Selank can be switched out with N-Acetyl Semax after 6 weeks to continue with the cycle without desensitization

N-Acetyl Selank + BPC-157 + TB-4

Overview

- Selank was created from Tuftsin (a peptide that naturally comes from the antibody immunoglobulin G) with additional sequins to enhance the peptides' stability

- N-Acetyl Selank (added amide group) is better absorbed, more potent, and has a longer half-life than Selank

- BPC-157 stands for body-protective compound. It was discovered in the human gastric juice

- Thymosin Beta-4 (TB-4) is related to thymosin, a hormone secreted by your thymus, with its primary function to produce T cells, which is an essential aspect of the immune system.

Why Add These Together?

- Selank works by regulating neurotransmitter levels in the brain, including serotonin, dopamine, and GABA. Additionally, Selank enhances BDNF while reducing pain, inflammation, and cancerous development

- BPC-157 is neuroprotective (brain), cardioprotective (heart), gastroprotective (stomach), and musculoskeletal protective (joints, ligaments and muscles).

- Thymosin Beta-4 works by binding to actin, which is a protein that influences the action and formation of most cells in our body. Enhancing the mechanism of actin, leads to faster healing time, especially in injured areas

- BPC-157 & TB-4 are often paired together to treat TBIs and concussions

- Combining these peptides enhances learning, memory, and mood with additional full-body healing and protective benefits, especially regarding the brain

Research Benefits

Benefits

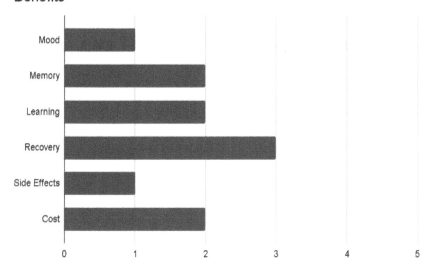

- Neuroprotective (brain), cardioprotective (heart), gastroprotective (stomach), and musculoskeletal protective (joints, ligaments and muscles)

- Increases BDNF

- Increases dopamine and serotonin signaling

- It can be used to help treat generalized anxiety disorder

- Enhanced learning and memory capacity

- Promotes healthy relaxation by increasing GABA

- Helps balance sleep vs. wakefulness

- Helps regulate inflammation and has anti-viral properties

Research Side Effects

- Redness, itchiness, and swelling of injection sites

- Water retention

- Excess and prolonged use of Selank can lead to desensitization

- Temporary tiredness

Matthew's Personal Insight on Research Dosing

- N-Acetyl Selank

    ¤ 100-300 mcg through a subcutaneous injection

    ¤ 750-1000 mcg through an intranasal spray (preferred method)

- BPC-157

    ¤ 400-600 mcg per injection

- TB-4

    ¤ 300 mcg to 1-gram subcutaneous injection

Matthew's Personal Insight on Research Cycling

- N-Acetyl Selank

    ¤ 6 weeks on, 6 weeks off

- BPC-157, TB-4

    ¤ Intended to take a 6-week cycle of Selank

- Best to take this peptide combo in the morning to prevent sleep disturbances

- These can all be taken through an intranasal spray

Matthew's Opinion

- This is a great peptide combo if the main goal is to help with healing the brain

- TB-4 and BPC-157 pack a powerful brain healing aspect to this stack, which is why they're often used to treat TBIs and concussions

- I like how all of these peptides can be taken through an intranasal spray or injecting

- N-Acetyl Selank can be switched out with N-Acetyl Semax after 6 weeks to continue with the cycle without desensitization

N-Acetyl Selank + BPC-157 + TB-4 + Cerebrolysin

Overview

- Selank was created from Tuftsin (a peptide that naturally comes from the antibody immunoglobulin G) with additional sequins to enhance the peptides' stability

- N-Acetyl Selank (added amide group) is better absorbed, more potent, and has a longer half-life than Selank

- BPC-157 stands for body-protective compound. It was discovered in the human gastric juice

- Thymosin Beta-4 (TB-4) is related to thymosin, a hormone that is secreted by your thymus, with its main function to produce T cells, which is an essential aspect of the immune system

- Cerebrolysin is a neuropeptide that comes from young pig brains

Why Add These Together?

- Selank works by regulating neurotransmitter levels in the brain, including serotonin, dopamine, and GABA. Additionally, Selank enhances BDNF while reducing pain, inflammation, and cancerous development

- BPC-157 is neuroprotective (brain), cardioprotective (heart), gastroprotective (stomach), and musculoskeletal protective (joints, ligaments and muscles).

- Thymosin Beta-4 works by binding to actin, which is a protein that influences the action and formation of most cells in the body. Enhancing the mechanism of actin leads to faster healing time, especially in injured areas

- BPC-157 & TB-4 are often paired together to treat TBIs and concussions

- Cerebrolysin contains:

  - ¤ Nerve growth factors (promotes nerve regeneration)

  - ¤ BDFN (enhances growth of neurons)

  - ¤ P-21 (enhances DNA repair process)

  - ¤ Enkephalins (reduces pain, inflammation and cancerous growth)

  - ¤ Orexin (improves learning, memory and circadian rhythm health)

- Combining these peptides greatly enhances learning, memory, and mood with additional full-body healing and protective benefits, especially regarding the brain

Research Benefits

Benefits

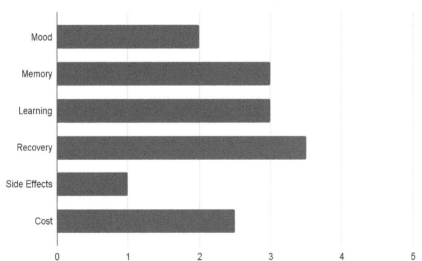

- Neuroprotective (brain), cardioprotective (heart), gastroprotective (stomach), and musculoskeletal protective (joints, ligaments and muscles)

- Increases BDNF

- Helps treat concussions and TBI's

- Increases dopamine and serotonin signaling

- It can be used to help treat generalized anxiety disorder

- Enhanced learning and memory capacity

- Promotes healthy relaxation by increasing GABA

- Helps balance sleep vs wakefulness

- Helps regulate inflammation and has anti-viral properties

Research Side Effects

- Redness, itchiness, and swelling of injection sites

- Water retention

- Excess and prolonged use of Selank can lead to desensitization

- Temporary tiredness

- Headache

- Nausea

Matthew's Personal Insight on Research Dosing

- N-Acetyl Selank

  ¤ 100-300 mcg through a subcutaneous injection

  ¤ 750-1000 mcg through an intranasal spray (preferred method)

- BPC-157

  - ¤ 400-600 mcg per injection

- TB-4

  - ¤ 300 mcg to 1-gram subcutaneous injection

- Cerebrolysin

  - ¤ 5-10 ml (215 mg/ml) through a subcutaneous injection

Matthew's Personal Insight on Research Cycling

- N-Acetyl Selank

  - ¤ 6 weeks on, 6 weeks off

- BPC-157, TB-4

  - ¤ Intended to take a 6-week cycle of Selank

- Cerebrolysin

  - ¤ 10–20-day cycles

  - ¤ Dosing intensity and frequency will vary with conditions

- Best to take this peptide combo in the morning to prevent sleep disturbances

Matthew's Opinion

- This would be my go-to peptide combo to heal any TBIs or concussions.

- TB-4 and BPC-157 pack a powerful brain healing aspect to this stack, which is why they're often used to treat TBIs and concussions

- Cerebrolysin is one of my favorite neuropeptides as it contains several powerful neuroactive compounds with a high safety profile

- N-Acetyl Selank can be switched out with N-Acetyl Semax after 6 weeks to continue with the cycle without desensitization

N-Acetyl Selank + BPC-157 + TB-4 + Cerebrolysin + PE-22-88

Overview

- Selank was created from Tuftsin (a peptide that naturally comes from the antibody immunoglobulin G) with additional sequins to enhance the peptides' stability

- N-Acetyl Selank (added amide group) is better absorbed, more potent, and has a longer half-life than Selank

- BPC-157 stands for body-protective compound. It was discovered in the human gastric juice

- Thymosin Beta-4 (TB-4) is related to thymosin, a hormone that is secreted by your thymus, with its main function to produce T cells, which is an essential aspect of the immune system

- Cerebrolysin is a neuropeptide that comes from young pig brains

- PE-22-28 is a peptide derived from Spadin (a natural antidepressant peptide found in human blood)

Why Add These Together?

- Selank works by regulating neurotransmitter levels in the brain, including serotonin, dopamine, and GABA. Additionally, Selank enhances BDNF while reducing pain, inflammation, and cancerous development

- BPC-157 is neuroprotective (brain), cardioprotective (heart), gastroprotective (stomach), and musculoskeletal protective (joints, ligaments and muscles).

- Thymosin Beta-4 works by binding to actin, which is a protein that influences the action and formation of most cells in the body.

307

Enhancing the mechanism of actin, leads to faster healing time, especially in injured areas

- BPC-157 & TB-4 are often paired together to treat TBIs and concussions

- Cerebrolysin contains:

  ¤ Nerve growth factors (promotes nerve regeneration)

  ¤ BDFN (enhances growth of neurons)

  ¤ P-21 (enhances DNA repair process)

  ¤ Enkephalins (reduces pain, inflammation and cancerous growth)

  ¤ Orexin (improves learning, memory and circadian rhythm health)

- PE-22-28 binds to TREK-1 receptors in the brain. Blocking the TREK-1 channel. By reducing the levels of TREK-1, the body has a heightened ability to manage stress, memory recall, learning capabilities, and overall mood regulation

- Combining these peptides greatly enhances learning, memory, and mood with additional full-body healing and protective benefits, especially regarding the brain

Research Benefits

Benefits

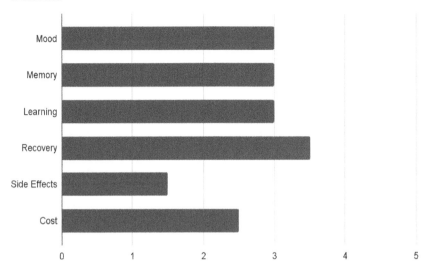

- Neuroprotective (brain), cardioprotective (heart), gastroprotective (stomach), and musculoskeletal protective (joints, ligaments and muscles)

- Increases BDNF

- Helps treat concussions and TBIs

- Increases dopamine and serotonin signaling

- It can be used to help treat generalized anxiety disorder

- Enhanced learning and memory capacity

- Promotes healthy relaxation by increasing GABA

- Helps balance sleep vs wakefulness

- Helps regulate inflammation and has anti-viral properties

Research Side Effects

- Redness, itchiness, and swelling of injection sites

- Water retention

- Excess and prolonged use of Selank can lead to desensitization

- Temporary tiredness

- Headache

- Nausea

Matthew's Personal Insight on Research Dosing

- N-Acetyl Selank

  - 100-300 mcg through a subcutaneous injection

  - 750-1000 mcg through an intranasal spray (preferred method)

- PE-22-88

  - 400 mcg intranasally

- BPC-157

  - 400-600 mcg per injection

- TB-4

  - 300 mcg to 1-gram subcutaneous injection

- Cerebrolysin

  - 5-10 ml (215 mg/ml) through a subcutaneous injection

Matthew's Personal Insight on Research Cycling

- N-Acetyl Selank

  ¤ 6 weeks on, 6 weeks off

- BPC-157, TB-4, PE-22-88

  ¤ Intended to take a 6-week cycle of Selank

- Cerebrolysin

  ¤ 10–20-day cycles

  ¤ Dosing intensity and frequency will vary with the conditions

- Best to take this peptide combo in the morning to prevent sleep disturbances

- All of these peptides can be taken through an intranasal spray

Matthew's Opinion

- Cerebrolysin is one of my favorite neuropeptides as it contains several powerful neuroactive compounds with a high safety profile

- PE-22-88 is a nice addition to this stack to add to mood enhancement. Overall, this peptide is much more natural and safer than pharmaceutical antidepressants

- TB-4 and BPC-157 pack a powerful brain healing aspect to this stack, which is why they're often used to treat TBIs and concussions

- I like how these peptides can be taken through an intranasal spray or injecting.

- N-Acetyl Selank can be switched out with N-Acetyl Semax after 6 weeks to continue with the cycle without desensitization

N-Acetyl Selank + BPC-157 + TB-4 + Cerebrolysin + PE-22-88 + MOD-GRF-1-29 + Ipamorelin

Overview

- Selank was created from Tuftsin (a peptide that naturally comes from the antibody immunoglobulin G) with additional sequins to enhance the peptides' stability

- N-Acetyl Selank (added amide group) is better absorbed, more potent, and has a longer half-life than Selank

- BPC-157 stands for body-protective compound. It was discovered in the human gastric juice

- PE-22-28 is a peptide derived from Spadin (a natural antidepressant peptide found in human blood)

- Thymosin Beta-4 (TB-4) is related to thymosin, a hormone that is secreted by your thymus, with its main function to produce T cells, which is an essential aspect of the immune system

- Cerebrolysin is a neuropeptide that comes from young pig brains

- MOD-GRF-1-29 is a GHRH (Growth Hormone Releasing Hormone)

- Ipamorelin is the mildest of GHRPs (Growth Hormone Releasing Peptide)

Why Add These Together?

- Selank works by regulating neurotransmitter levels in the brain, including serotonin, dopamine, and GABA. Additionally, Selank enhances BDNF while reducing pain, inflammation, and cancerous development

312

- BPC-157 is neuroprotective (brain), cardioprotective (heart), gastroprotective (stomach), and musculoskeletal protective (joints, ligaments and muscles).

- Thymosin Beta-4 works by binding to actin, which is a protein that influences the action and formation of most cells in our body. Enhancing the mechanism of actin, leads to faster healing time, especially in injured areas

- BPC-157 & TB-4 are often paired together to treat TBIs and concussions

- MOD-GRF-1-29 goes up to the anterior pituitary gland and signals the body to create growth hormone

- Ipamorelin works by inhibiting somatostatin on the hypothalamus to allow the release of growth hormone

- Cerebrolysin contains:

  ¤ Nerve growth factors (promotes nerve regeneration)

  ¤ BDFN (enhances growth of neurons)

  ¤ P-21 (enhances DNA repair process)

  ¤ Enkephalins (reduces pain, inflammation and cancerous growth)

  ¤ Orexin (improves learning, memory and circadian rhythm health)

- PE-22-28 binds to TREK-1 receptors in the brain. Blocking the TREK-1 channel. By reducing the levels of TREK-1, the body has a heightened ability to manage stress, memory recall, learning capabilities, and overall mood regulation

- Combining these peptides ensures the creation and release of growth hormone occurs simultaneously, greatly enhancing learning, memory, and mood with additional full-body healing and protective benefits, especially regarding the brain

Research Benefits

Benefits

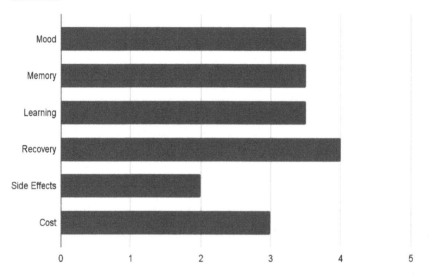

- Neuroprotective (brain), cardioprotective (heart), gastroprotective (stomach), and musculoskeletal protective (joints, ligaments and muscles)

- Increases BDNF

- Helps treat concussions and TBI's

- Increases dopamine and serotonin signaling

- Increase in the creation and release of endogenous growth hormone

- Accelerates wound healing

- Promotes muscle growth

- Enhanced learning and memory capacity

- Promotes healthy relaxation by increasing GABA

- Helps regulate inflammation and has anti-viral properties

Research Side Effects

- Redness, itchiness, and swelling of injection sites

- Water retention

- Excess and prolonged use of Selank can lead to desensitization

- Temporary tiredness

- Headache

- Nausea

Matthew's Personal Insight on Research Dosing

- N-Acetyl Selank

  - 100-300 mcg through a subcutaneous injection

  - 750-1000 mcg through an intranasal spray (preferred method)

- PE-22-88

  - 400 mcg intranasally

- BPC-157

  - 400-600 mcg per injection

- MOD-GRF-1-29

  - 100 mcg per injection (more is not better)

- Ipamorelin

  - 100-300 mcg per injection

- TB-4

  ¤ 300 mcg to 1-gram subcutaneous injection

- Cerebrolysin

  ¤ 5-10 ml (215 mg/ml) through a subcutaneous injection

Matthew's Personal Insight on Research Cycling

- N-Acetyl Selank

  ¤ 6 weeks on, 6 weeks off

- BPC-157, TB-4, PE-22-88, Ipamorelin, MOD-GRF-1-29

  ¤ Intended to take with 6-week cycle of Selank

- Cerebrolysin

  ¤ 10–20-day cycles

  ¤ Dosing intensity and frequency will vary with the conditions

- Ipamorelin, MOD-GRF-1-29

  ¤ Carbohydrates and fatty acids can blunt growth hormone release. Best taken 30 minutes before eating or 2 hours after eating

- Best to take this peptide combo in the morning to prevent sleep disturbances

Matthew's Opinion

- Ipamorelin and MOD-GRF-1-29 is one of my favorite peptide combos for increasing endogenous growth hormone that I have used for several years on and off. Adding this enhances the full-body healing, anti-aging, and performance benefits of this stack

- Cerebrolysin is one of my favorite neuropeptides as it contains several powerful neuroactive compounds with a high safety profile

- PE-22-88 is nice addition to this stack to add to mood enhancement. Overall, this peptide is much more natural and safer than pharmaceutical antidepressants

- TB-4 and BPC-157 pack a powerful brain healing aspect to this stack, which is why they're often used to treat TBIs and concussions

- I would take all of these through an injection to reduce the hassle of taking all of these peptides. And because MOD-GRF-1-29 and Ipamorelin cannot be taken through an intranasal spray

- N-Acetyl Selank can be switched out with N-Acetyl Semax after 6 weeks to continue with the cycle without desensitization

N-Acetyl Selank + BPC-157 + TB-4 + Cerebrolysin + PE-22-88 + Tesamorelin + Ipamorelin

Overview

- Selank was created from Tuftsin (a peptide that naturally comes from the antibody immunoglobulin G) with additional sequins to enhance the peptides' stability

- N-Acetyl Selank (added amide group) is better absorbed, more potent, and has a longer half-life than Selank

- BPC-157 stands for body-protective compound. It was discovered in the human gastric juice

- PE-22-28 is a peptide derived from Spadin (a natural antidepressant peptide found in human blood)

- Thymosin Beta-4 (TB-4) is related to thymosin, a hormone that is secreted by your thymus, with its main function to produce T cells, which is an essential aspect of the immune system

- Cerebrolysin is a neuropeptide that comes from young pig brains

- Tesamorelin is a GHRH (Growth Hormone Releasing Hormone)

- Ipamorelin is the mildest of GHRP's (Growth Hormone Releasing Peptide)

Why Add These Together?

- Selank works by regulating neurotransmitter levels in the brain, including serotonin, dopamine, and GABA. Additionally, Selank enhances BDNF while reducing pain, inflammation, and cancerous development

- BPC-157 is neuroprotective (brain), cardioprotective (heart), gastroprotective (stomach), and musculoskeletal protective (joints, ligaments and muscles).

- Thymosin Beta-4 works by binding to actin, which is a protein that influences the action and formation of most cells in our body. Enhancing the mechanism of actin, leads to faster healing time, especially in injured areas

- BPC-157 & TB-4 are often paired together to treat TBIs and concussions

- Tesamorelin goes up to the anterior pituitary gland and signals the body to create growth hormone (Stronger than MOD-GRF-1-29)

- Ipamorelin works by inhibiting somatostatin on the hypothalamus to allow the release of growth hormone

- Cerebrolysin contains:

  ¤ Nerve growth factors (promotes nerve regeneration)

  ¤ BDFN (enhances growth of neurons)

  ¤ P-21 (enhances DNA repair process)

  ¤ Enkephalins (reduces pain, inflammation and cancerous growth)

  ¤ Orexin (improves learning, memory and circadian rhythm health)

- PE-22-28 binds to TREK-1 receptors in the brain. Blocking the TREK-1 channel. By reducing the levels of TREK-1, the body has a heightened ability to manage stress, memory recall, learning capabilities, and overall mood regulation

- Combining these peptides ensures the creation and release of growth hormone occurs simultaneously, greatly enhancing learning, memory, and mood with additional full-body healing and protective benefits, especially regarding the brain

Research Benefits

Benefits

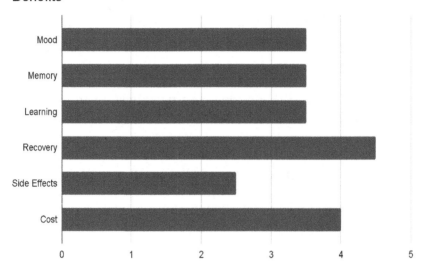

- Neuroprotective (brain), cardioprotective (heart), gastroprotective (stomach), and musculoskeletal protective (joints, ligaments and muscles)

- Increases BDNF

- Helps treat concussions and TBIs

- Increase in the creation and release of endogenous growth hormone

- Accelerates wound healing

- Promotes muscle growth

- Can be used to help treat generalized anxiety disorder

- Enhanced learning and memory capacity

- Promotes healthy relaxation by increasing GABA

- Helps regulate inflammation and has anti-viral properties

Research Side Effects

- Redness, itchiness, and swelling of injection sites

- Water retention

- Excess and prolonged use of Selank can lead to desensitization

- Temporary tiredness

- Headache

- Nausea

- Sharp increase in IGF-1 levels

Matthew's Personal Insight on Research Dosing

- N-Acetyl Selank

  - 100-300 mcg through a subcutaneous injection

  - 750-1000 mcg through an intranasal spray (preferred method)

- PE-22-88

  - 400 mcg intranasally

- BPC-157

  - 400-600 mcg per injection

- Tesamorelin

  - 500-2000 mcg per injection

- Ipamorelin

  - 100-300 mcg per injection

- TB-4

  ¤ 300 mcg to 1-gram subcutaneous injection

- Cerebrolysin

  ¤ 5-10 ml (215 mg/ml) through a subcutaneous injection

Matthew's Personal Insight on Research Cycling

- N-Acetyl Selank

  ¤ 6 weeks on, 6 weeks off

- BPC-157, TB-4, PE-22-88, Ipamorelin, Tesamorelin

  ¤ Intended to take daily with a 6-week cycle of Selank

- Cerebrolysin

  ¤ 10–20-day cycles

  ¤ Dosing intensity and frequency will vary with the conditions

- Ipamorelin, Tesamorelin

  ¤ Carbohydrates and fatty acids can blunt growth hormone release. Best taken 30 minutes before eating or 2 hours after eating

- Best to take this peptide combo in the morning to prevent sleep disturbances

Matthew's Opinion

- Ipamorelin and Tesamorelin is the "gold standard" combo for increasing endogenous growth hormone. Adding this enhances the full-body healing, anti-aging, and performance benefits of this stack

- Cerebrolysin is one of my favorite neuropeptides as it contains several powerful neuroactive compounds with a high safety profile

- PE-22-88 is nice addition to this stack to add to mood enhancement. Overall, this peptide is much more natural and safer than pharmaceutical antidepressants.

- TB-4 and BPC-157 pack a powerful brain healing aspect to this stack, which is why they're often used to treat TBIs and concussions

- I would take all of these through an injection to reduce the hassle of taking all of these peptides. And because Tesamorelin and Ipamorelin cannot be taken through an intranasal spray

- N-Acetyl Selank can be switched out with N-Acetyl Semax after 6 weeks to continue with the cycle without desensitization

N-Acetyl Selank + BPC-157 + TB-4 + Cerebrolysin + PE-22-88 + Tesamorelin + Ipamorelin + FGL(L)

Overview

- Selank was created from Tuftsin (a peptide that naturally comes from the antibody immunoglobulin G) with additional sequins to enhance the peptides' stability

- N-Acetyl Selank (added amide group) is better absorbed, more potent, and has a longer half-life than Selank

- BPC-157 stands for body-protective compound. It was discovered in the human gastric juice

- PE-22-28 is a peptide derived from Spadin (a natural antidepressant peptide found in human blood)

- FGL(L) is a variant of the Neural Cell Adhesion Molecule (NCAM), which is found naturally on the surface of nerve cells (neurons) and glial cells (protect neurons

- Thymosin Beta-4 (TB-4) is related to thymosin, a hormone that is secreted by your thymus, with its main function to produce T cells, which is an essential aspect of the immune system

- Cerebrolysin is a neuropeptide that comes from young pig brains

- Tesamorelin is a GHRH (Growth Hormone Releasing Hormone)

- Ipamorelin is the mildest of GHRP's (Growth Hormone Releasing Peptide)

Why Add These Together?

- Selank works by regulating neurotransmitter levels in the brain, including serotonin, dopamine, and GABA. Additionally, Selank enhances BDNF while reducing pain, inflammation, and cancerous development

- BPC-157 is neuroprotective (brain), cardioprotective (heart), gastroprotective (stomach), and musculoskeletal protective (joints, ligaments and muscles).

- Thymosin Beta-4 works by binding to actin, which is a protein that influences the action and formation of most cells in our body. Enhancing the mechanism of actin, leads to faster healing time, especially in injured areas

- BPC-157 & TB-4 are often paired together to treat TBIs and concussions

- Tesamorelin goes up to the anterior pituitary gland and signals the body to create growth hormone (Stronger than MOD-GRF-1-29)

- Ipamorelin works by inhibiting somatostatin on the hypothalamus to allow the release of growth hormone

- Cerebrolysin contains:

  ¤ Nerve growth factors (promotes nerve regeneration)

  ¤ BDFN (enhances growth of neurons)

  ¤ P-21 (enhances DNA repair process)

  ¤ Enkephalins (reduces pain, inflammation and cancerous growth)

  ¤ Orexin (improves learning, memory and circadian rhythm health)

- PE-22-28 binds to TREK-1 receptors in the brain. Blocking the TREK-1 channel. By reducing the levels of TREK-1, the body has a heightened ability to manage stress, memory recall, learning capabilities, and overall mood regulation

- FGL directly increases fibroblast growth factor receptors, which increases neuronal growth and survival

- Combining these peptides ensures the creation and release of growth hormone occurs simultaneously, greatly enhancing learning, memory, and mood with additional full-body healing and protective benefits, especially regarding the brain

Research Benefits

Benefits

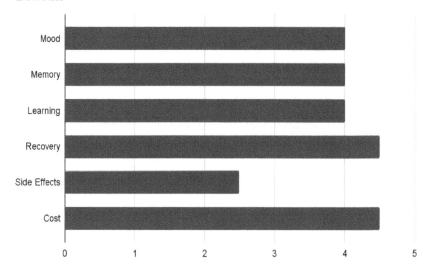

- Neuroprotective (brain), cardioprotective (heart), gastroprotective (stomach), and musculoskeletal protective (joints, ligaments and muscles)

- Increases BDNF

- Helps treat concussions and TBIs

- Increase in the creation and release of endogenous growth hormone

- Accelerates wound healing

- Promotes muscle growth

- Can be used to help treat generalized anxiety disorder

- Enhanced learning and memory capacity

- Promotes healthy relaxation by increasing GABA

- Helps regulate inflammation and has anti-viral properties

Research Side Effects

- Redness, itchiness, and swelling of injection sites

- Water retention

- Excess and prolonged use of Selank can lead to desensitization

- Temporary tiredness

- Headache

- Nausea

- Sharp increase in IGF-1 levels

Matthew's Personal Insight on Research Dosing

- N-Acetyl Selank

  - 100-300 mcg through a subcutaneous injection

  - 750-1000 mcg through an intranasal spray (preferred method)

- PE-22-88

  - 400 mcg intranasally

- BPC-157

  ¤ 400-600 mcg per injection

- FGL(L)

  ¤ 1-2 mg per subcutaneous injection

  ¤ Younger subjects in their 30's are recommended do a lower dose (1mg or less)

- Tesamorelin

  ¤ 500-2000 mcg per injection

- Ipamorelin

  ¤ 100-300 mcg per injection

- TB-4

  ¤ 300 mcg to 1-gram subcutaneous injection

- Cerebrolysin

  ¤ 5-10 ml (215 mg/ml) through a subcutaneous injection

Matthew's Personal Insight on Research Cycling

- N-Acetyl Selank

  ¤ 6 weeks on, 6 weeks off

- BPC-157, TB-4, PE-22-88, Ipamorelin, Tesamorelin, FGL(L)

  ¤ Intended to take daily with a 6-week cycle of Selank

- Cerebrolysin

  ¤ 10–20-day cycles

  ¤ Dosing intensity and frequency will vary with the conditions

- Ipamorelin, Tesamorelin

    - ¤ Carbohydrates and fatty acids can blunt growth hormone release. Best taken 30 minutes before eating or 2 hours after eating

- Best to take this peptide combo in the morning to prevent sleep disturbances

Matthew's Opinion

- Ipamorelin and Tesamorelin is the "gold standard" combo for increasing endogenous growth hormone. Adding this enhances the full-body healing, anti-aging, and performance benefits of this stack

- Cerebrolysin is one of my favorite neuropeptides as it contains several powerful neuroactive compounds with a high safety profile

- PE-22-88 is an excellent addition to this stack to add to mood enhancement. Overall, this peptide is much more natural and safer than pharmaceutical antidepressants

- FGL(L) gives the body more brain-building blocks and then helps connect them (that's how I think about it)

- TB-4 and BPC-157 pack a powerful brain healing aspect to this stack, which is why they're often used to treat TBI's and concussions

- I would take all of these through an injection to reduce the hassle of taking all of these peptides. And because Tesamorelin and Ipamorelin cannot be taken through an intranasal spray

- N-Acetyl Selank can be switched out with N-Acetyl Semax after 6 weeks to continue with the cycle without desensitization. I would recommend using this protocol in periods of 6 weeks on and 6 weeks off, regardless of switching out to Semax

N-Acetyl Selank + BPC-157 + TB-4 + Cerebrolysin + PE-22-88 + Tesamorelin + Ipamorelin + FGL(L) + Dihexa

Overview

- Selank was created from Tuftsin (a peptide that naturally comes from the antibody immunoglobulin G) with additional sequins to enhance the peptides' stability

- N-Acetyl Selank (added amide group) is better absorbed, more potent, and has a longer half-life than Selank

- BPC-157 stands for body-protective compound. It was discovered in the human gastric juice

- PE-22-28 is a peptide derived from Spadin (a natural antidepressant peptide found in human blood)

- FGL(L) is a variant of the Neural Cell Adhesion Molecule (NCAM), which is found naturally on the surface of nerve cells (neurons) and glial cells (protect neurons)

- Thymosin Beta-4 (TB-4) is related to thymosin, a hormone that is secreted by your thymus, with its main function to produce T cells, which is an essential aspect of the immune system

- Cerebrolysin is a neuropeptide that comes from young pig brains

- Tesamorelin is a GHRH (Growth Hormone Releasing Hormone)

- Ipamorelin is the mildest of GHRPs (Growth Hormone Releasing Peptide)

- Dihexa was initially derived from angiotensin IV (a hormone naturally produced in our body that helps with memory)

Why Add These Together?

- Selank works by regulating neurotransmitter levels in the brain, including serotonin, dopamine, and GABA. Additionally, Selank enhances BDNF while reducing pain, inflammation, and cancerous development

- BPC-157 is neuroprotective (brain), cardioprotective (heart), gastroprotective (stomach), and musculoskeletal protective (joints, ligaments and muscles).

- Thymosin Beta-4 works by binding to actin, which is a protein that influences the action and formation of most cells in our body. Enhancing the mechanism of actin, leads to faster healing time, especially in injured areas

- BPC-157 & TB-4 are often paired together to treat TBIs and concussions

- Tesamorelin goes up to the anterior pituitary gland and signals the body to create growth hormone (Stronger than MOD-GRF-1-29)

- Ipamorelin works by inhibiting somatostatin on the hypothalamus to allow the release of growth hormone

- Cerebrolysin contains:

  ¤ Nerve growth factors (promotes nerve regeneration)

  ¤ BDFN (enhances growth of neurons)

  ¤ P-21 (enhances DNA repair process)

  ¤ Enkephalins (reduces pain, inflammation and cancerous growth)

  ¤ Orexin (improves learning, memory and circadian rhythm health)

- PE-22-28 binds to TREK-1 receptors in the brain. Blocking the TREK-1 channel. By reducing the levels of TREK-1, the body has a heightened ability to manage stress, memory recall, learning capabilities, and overall mood regulation

- FGL directly increases fibroblast growth factor receptors, which increases neuronal growth and survival

- Dihexa has been reported to be 7x more potent than brain-derived-neurotrophic factor (BDFN), which has a multitude of benefits for the brain and body

- Combining these peptides ensures the creation and release of growth hormone occurs simultaneously, greatly enhancing learning, memory, and mood with additional full-body healing and protective benefits, especially regarding the brain

Research Benefits

Benefits

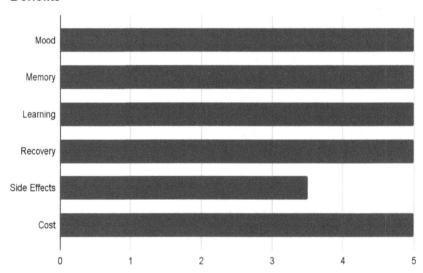

- Neuroprotective (brain), cardioprotective (heart), gastroprotective (stomach), and musculoskeletal protective (joints, ligaments and muscles)

- Increases BDNF

- Helps treat concussions and TBIs

- Increase in the creation and release of endogenous growth hormone

- Accelerates wound healing

- Promotes muscle growth

- It can be used to help treat generalized anxiety disorder

- Enhanced learning and memory capacity

- Promotes healthy relaxation by increasing GABA

- Helps regulate inflammation and has anti-viral properties

Research Side Effects

- Redness, itchiness, and swelling of injection sites

- Water retention

- Excess and prolonged use of Selank can lead to desensitization

- Temporary tiredness

- Headache

- Nausea

- A sharp increase in IGF-1 levels

- Mood swings

- Insomnia

Matthew's Personal Insight on Research Dosing

- N-Acetyl Selank

  - 100-300 mcg through a subcutaneous injection

  - 750-1000 mcg through an intranasal spray (preferred method)

- PE-22-88

  - 400 mcg intranasally

- BPC-157

  - 400-600 mcg per injection

- FGL(L)

  - 1-2 mg per subcutaneous injection

  - Younger subjects in their 30s are recommended to do a lower dose (1mg or less)

- Tesamorelin

  - 500-2000 mcg per injection

- Ipamorelin

  - 100-300 mcg per injection

- TB-4

  - 300 mcg to 1-gram subcutaneous injection

- Dihexa

  - 10-50 mg taken daily either through powder or as a cream (rub onto inner forearms)

- Cerebrolysin

⌑ 5-10 ml (215 mg/ml) through a subcutaneous injection

Matthew's Personal Insight on Research Cycling

- N-Acetyl Selank

  ⌑ 6 weeks on, 6 weeks off

- BPC-157, TB-4, PE-22-88, Ipamorelin, Tesamorelin, FGL(L), Dihexa

  ⌑ Intended to take daily with a 6-week cycle of Selank

- Cerebrolysin

  ⌑ 10–20-day cycles

  ⌑ Dosing intensity and frequency will vary with the conditions

- Ipamorelin, Tesamorelin

  ⌑ Carbohydrates and fatty acids can blunt growth hormone release. Best taken 30 minutes before eating or 2 hours after eating

- Best to take this peptide combo in the morning to prevent sleep disturbance

Matthew's Opinion

- Ipamorelin and Tesamorelin is the "gold standard" combo for increasing endogenous growth hormone. Adding this enhances the full-body healing, anti-aging, and performance benefits of this stack

- Cerebrolysin is one of my favorite neuropeptides as it contains several powerful neuroactive compounds with a high safety profile

- PE-22-88 is an excellent addition to this stack to add to mood enhancement. Overall, this peptide is much more natural and safer than pharmaceutical antidepressants

- It is wild how Dihexa has been reported to be 7x more potent than brain-derived-neurotrophic factor (BDFN). This dramatically adds to the brain-boosting benefits of this protocol

- I would start at the lower dosing and frequency scheme (1-3x week, 10 mg) by taking Dihexa since it is a potent neuropeptide with a long half-life (7-10 days), and this stack already has multiple brain-boosting peptides.

- FGL(L) gives the body more brain-building blocks and then helps connect them (that's how I think about it)

- TB-4 and BPC-157 pack a powerful brain healing aspect to this stack, which is why they're often used to treat TBIs and concussions

- I would take all of these through an injection to reduce the hassle of taking all of these peptides besides Dihexa (which must be taken orally or through a cream). And because Tesamorelin and Ipamorelin cannot be taken through an intranasal spray

- N-Acetyl Selank can be switched out with N-Acetyl Semax after 6 weeks to continue the cycle without desensitization. I would recommend using this protocol in periods of 6 weeks on and 6 weeks off, regardless of switching to Semax

14. Peptides Combos for Cosmetics

MOD-GRF-1-29 + Ipamorelin

Overview

- MOD-GRF-1-29 is a GHRH (Growth Hormone Releasing Hormone)

- Ipamorelin is the mildest of GHRPs (Growth Hormone Releasing Peptide)

- This is one of the most commonly stacked GH peptides

Why Add These Together?

- MOD-GRF-1-29 goes up to the anterior pituitary gland and signals the body to create growth hormone

- Ipamorelin works by inhibiting somatostatin on the hypothalamus to allow the release of growth hormone

- Combining these peptides ensures the creation and release of growth hormone occurs simultaneously

Research Benefits

Benefits

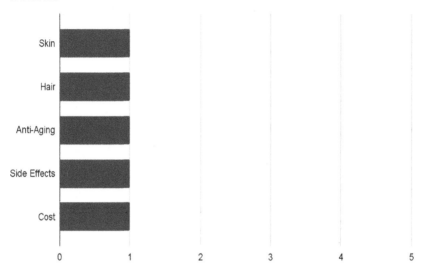

- Increase in the creation and release of endogenous growth hormone

- Promotes muscle growth

- Helps with mood and stress resilience

- Slows down aging

- Improves sleep

- Promotes a balanced inflammatory response

- Improves bone density

Research Side Effects

- Redness, itchiness, and swelling of injection sites

- Water retention

- Facial flushing

Matthew's Personal Insight on Research Dosing & Cycling

- MOD-GRF-1-29

  - 100 mcg per injection (more is not better)

- Ipamorelin

  - 100-300 mcg per injection

- Multiple injections can be given a day to increase GH secretion. Often used in bodybuilding

- 5 days on, 2 days off, 10-12 weeks on, 4-8 weeks off

- Carbohydrates and fatty acids can blunt growth hormone release. Best taken 30 minutes before eating or 2 hours after eating

Matthew's Personal Insight on Research Timing & Benefits

- Burning Fat

  - Before a workout in a fasted state

- Building Muscle

  - After a workout in a fasted state

- Sleep

  - Before bed in a fasted state

- General Anti-Aging

  - In the morning in a fasted state

Matthew's Opinion

- This is one of my favorite peptide combos that I have used for several years on and off

- Since it offers many benefits, I have placed this combo in several peptide combo categories.

- This creates an endogenous growth hormone increase while having a high safety profile. Growth hormone is the hormone of "vitality," making this a great beginner stack for cosmetic enhancement

MOD-GRF-1-29 + Ipamorelin + GHK-Cu

Overview

- MOD-GRF-1-29 is a GHRH (Growth Hormone Releasing Hormone)

- Ipamorelin is the mildest of GHRPs (Growth Hormone Releasing Peptide)

- GHK-Cu is a naturally occurring copper peptide found in human plasma. As people age, they naturally lose the ability to produce this

Why Add These Together?

- MOD-GRF-1-29 goes up to the anterior pituitary gland and signals the body to create growth hormone

- Ipamorelin works by inhibiting somatostatin on the hypothalamus to allow the release of growth hormone

- GHK-Cu increases collagen, stem cell production, and bone formation by stimulating chondrocytes in bones. GHK-Cu blocks the release of oxidative damage and enhances angiogenesis (development of new blood cells)

- Combining these peptides ensures the creation and release of growth hormone occur simultaneously while adding multiple anti-aging and cosmetic enhancing benefits

Research Benefits

Benefits

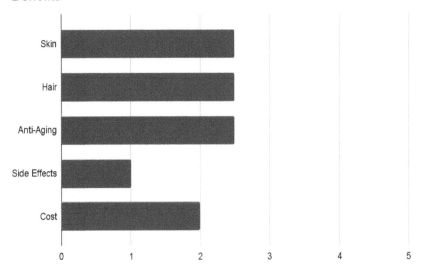

- Increase in the creation and release of endogenous growth hormone

- Promotes muscle growth

- Helps with mood and stress resilience

- Slows down aging

- Improves sleep

- Tightens loose skin and enhances skin elasticity

- Promotes hair growth

- Improves bone density

Research Side Effects

- Redness, itchiness, and swelling of injection sites

- Water retention

- Facial flushing

- Possibility for copper toxicity

Matthew's Personal Insight on Research Dosing

- MOD-GRF-1-29

    ¤ 100 mcg per injection (more is not better)

- Ipamorelin

    ¤ 100-300 mcg per injection

- GHK-Cu

    ¤ For subcutaneous injections: 1-2 mg per day

    ¤ For topical: apply to the area of healing

    ¤ For hair: micro-needle after a shower before applying

Matthew's Personal Insight on Research Cycling

- MOD-GRF-1-29, Ipamorelin

    ¤ Multiple injections can be given a day to increase GH secretion. Often used in bodybuilding

    ¤ 5 days on, 2 days off, 10-12 weeks on, 4-8 weeks off

    ¤ Carbohydrates and fatty acids can blunt growth hormone release. Best taken 30 minutes before eating or 2 hours after eating

- GHK-Cu

  - ¤ For subcutaneous injection

  - ¤ 6-week intervals

  - ¤ Can be cycled 3-4x a year

- For topical use

  - ¤ Continual use

Matthew's Personal Insight on Research Timing & Benefits - For Ipamorelin/MOD-GRF-1-29

- Burning Fat

  - ¤ Before a workout in a fasted state

- Building Muscle

  - ¤ After a workout in a fasted state

- Sleep

  - ¤ Before bed in a fasted state

- General Anti-Aging

  - ¤ In the morning in a fasted state

Matthew's Personal Insight on Research Timing & Benefits - GHK-Cu

- For Skin

  - ¤ Best to apply after micro-needling

- For Hair

- ¤ Best to apply after a shower. This will prevent the hair's natural oil from stopping GHK-Cu to be absorbed

- ¤ Absorption and hair growth can be enhanced by micro-needling before applying

Matthew's Opinion

- I have personally used this combo, and I have seen great benefit

- This combo takes time to see results (3-6 months)

- I would use GHK-Cu topically (skin and hair) and inject to get the most results

- It is important to micro-needle before applying topical GHK-Cu to get the most absorption and results

MOD-GRF-1-29 + Ipamorelin + GHK-Cu + PTD-DBM

Overview

- MOD-GRF-1-29 is a GHRH (Growth Hormone Releasing Hormone)

- Ipamorelin is the mildest of GHRPs (Growth Hormone Releasing Peptide)

- GHK-Cu is a naturally occurring copper peptide found in human plasma. As people age, they naturally lose the ability to produce this

- PTD-DBM is a topical man-made peptide to fight hair loss

Why Add These Together?

- MOD-GRF-1-29 goes up to the anterior pituitary gland and signals the body to create growth hormone

- Ipamorelin works by inhibiting somatostatin on the hypothalamus to allow the release of growth hormone

- GHK-Cu increases collagen, stem cell production, and bone formation by stimulating chondrocytes in bones. GHK-Cu blocks the release of oxidative damage and enhances angiogenesis (development of new blood cells)

- PTD-DBM both prevents hair loss and promotes the growth of new hair follicles by interfering with the CXXC5 protein binding

- Combining these peptides ensures the creation and release of growth hormone occurs simultaneously while adding multiple anti-aging and cosmetic enhancing benefits, especially in regards to hair growth

Research Benefits

Benefits

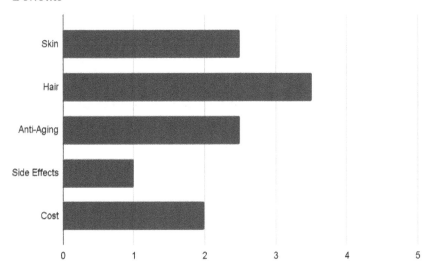

- Increase in the creation and release of endogenous growth hormone

- Promotes muscle growth

- Helps with mood and stress resilience

- Slows down aging

- Improves sleep

- Tightens loose skin and enhances skin elasticity

- Promotes hair growth

- Improves bone density

Research Side Effects

- Redness, itchiness, and swelling of injection sites

- Water retention

- Facial flushing

- Possibility for copper toxicity

Matthew's Personal Insight on Research Dosing

- MOD-GRF-1-29

  - ¤ 100 mcg per injection (more is not better)

- Ipamorelin

  - ¤ 100-300 mcg per injection

- GHK-Cu

  - ¤ For subcutaneous injections: 1-2 mg per day

  - ¤ For topical: apply to the area of healing

  - ¤ For hair: micro-needle after a shower before applying

- PTD-DBM

  - ¤ PTD-DBM sprays are usually available as a 0.001% solution in 25 ml of spray bottles

Matthew's Personal Insight on Research Cycling

- MOD-GRF-1-29, Ipamorelin

  - ¤ Multiple injections can be given a day to increase GH secretion. Often used in bodybuilding

  - ¤ 5 days on, 2 days off, 10-12 weeks on, 4-8 weeks off

- ¤ Carbohydrates and fatty acids can blunt growth hormone release. Best taken 30 minutes before eating or 2 hours after eating

- GHK-Cu

  - ¤ For subcutaneous injection

  - ¤ 6-week intervals

  - ¤ Can be cycled 3-4x a year

- For topical use

  - ¤ Continual use

- PTD-DBM

  - ¤ Use topical spray 1-2 a week

Matthew's Personal Insight on Research Timing & Benefits - For Ipamorelin/MOD-GRF-1-29

- Burning Fat

  - ¤ Before a workout in a fasted state

- Building Muscle

  - ¤ After a workout in a fasted state

- Sleep

  - ¤ Before bed in a fasted state

- General Anti-Aging

  - ¤ In the morning in a fasted state

Matthew's Personal Insight on Research Timing & Benefits - For GHK-Cu/PTD-DBM

- For Skin

  - ¤ Best to apply after micro-needling

- For Hair

  - ¤ Best to apply after a shower. This will prevent the hair's natural oil from stopping PTD-DBM and GHK-Cu to be absorbed

  - ¤ Absorption and hair growth can be enhanced by micro-needling before applying

  - ¤ Valproic acid is recommended to apply with PTD-DBM for maximal benefits

Matthew's Opinion

- I have been wanting to try PTD-DBM, as it seems promising and a great peptide to add to a cosmetic stack, especially if hair growth is the focus

- This combo takes time to see results (3-6 months)

- I would use GHK-Cu topically (skin and hair) and inject to get the most results

- It is important to micro-needle before applying topical GHK-Cu & PTD-DBM to get the most absorption and results

Tesamorelin + Ipamorelin + GHK-Cu + PTD-DBM

Overview

- Tesamorelin is a GHRH (Growth Hormone Releasing Hormone)

- Ipamorelin is the mildest of GHRPs (Growth Hormone Releasing Peptide)

- GHK-Cu is a naturally occurring copper peptide found in human plasma. As people age, they naturally lose the ability to produce this

- PTD-DBM is a topical man-made peptide to fight hair loss

Why Add These Together?

- Tesamorelin goes up to the anterior pituitary gland and signals the body to create growth hormone (Stronger than MOD-GRF-1-29)

- Ipamorelin works by inhibiting somatostatin on the hypothalamus to allow the release of growth hormone

- GHK-Cu increases collagen, stem cell production, and bone formation by stimulating chondrocytes in bones. GHK-Cu blocks the release of oxidative damage and enhances angiogenesis (development of new blood cells)

- PTD-DBM both prevents hair loss and promotes the growth of new hair follicles by interfering with the CXXC5 protein binding

- Combining these peptides ensures the creation and release of growth hormone occurs simultaneously while adding multiple anti-aging and cosmetic enhancing benefits, especially in regards to hair growth

Research Benefits

Benefits

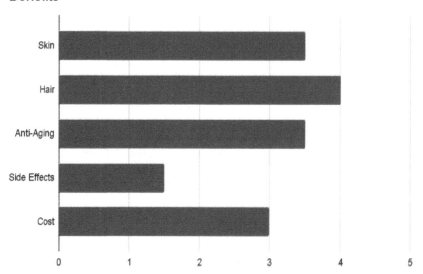

- Increase the creation and release of endogenous growth hormone

- Promotes muscle growth

- Helps with mood and stress resilience

- Slows down aging

- Improves sleep

- Tightens loose skin and enhances skin elasticity

- Promotes hair growth

- Improves bone density

Research Side Effects

- Redness, itchiness, and swelling of injection sites

- Water retention

- Facial flushing

- Possibility for copper toxicity

- A sharp increase in IGF-1 levels

Matthew's Personal Insight on ResearchDosing

- Tesamorelin

    ¤ 500-2000 mcg per injection

- Ipamorelin

    ¤ 100-300 mcg per injection

- GHK-Cu

    ¤ For subcutaneous injections: 1-2 mg per day

    ¤ For topical: apply to the area of healing

    ¤ For hair: micro-needle after a shower before applying

- PTD-DBM

    ¤ PTD-DBM sprays are usually available as a 0.001% solution in 25 ml of spray bottles

Matthew's Personal Insight on Research Cycling

- Tesamorelin, Ipamorelin

  - ¤ Multiple injections can be given a day to increase GH secretion. Often used in bodybuilding

  - ¤ 5 days on, 2 days off, 10-12 weeks on, 4-8 weeks off

  - ¤ Carbohydrates and fatty acids can blunt growth hormone release. Best taken 30 minutes before eating or 2 hours after eating

- GHK-Cu

  - ¤ For subcutaneous injection

  - ¤ 6-week intervals

  - ¤ Can be cycled 3-4x a year

- For topical use

  - ¤ Continual use

- PTD-DBM

  - ¤ Use topical spray 1-2 a week

Matthew's Personal Insight on Research Timing & Benefits - For Ipamorelin/Tesamorelin

- Burning Fat

  - ¤ Before a workout in a fasted state

- Building Muscle

  - ¤ After a workout in a fasted state

- Sleep

  ⌂ Before bed in a fasted state

- General Anti-Aging

  ⌂ In the morning in a fasted state

Matthew's Personal Insight on Research Timing & Benefits - For GHK-Cu/PTD-DBM

- For Skin

  ⌂ Best to apply after micro-needling

- For Hair

  ⌂ Best to apply after a shower. This will prevent the hair's natural oil from stopping PTD-DBM and GHK-Cu to be absorbed

  ⌂ Absorption and hair growth can be enhanced by micro-needling before applying

  ⌂ Valproic acid is recommended to apply with PTD-DBM for maximal benefits

Matthew's Opinion

- Ipamorelin and Tesamorelin is the gold standard peptide combo for increasing endogenous growth hormone, giving a nice boost in several cosmetic properties

- I have been wanting to try PTD-DBM, as it seems promising and a great peptide to add to a cosmetic stack, especially if hair growth is the focus

- This combo takes time to see results (3-6 months)

- I would use GHK-Cu topically (skin and hair) and inject to get the most results

- It is important to micro-needle before applying topical GHK-Cu & PTD-DBM to get the most absorption and results

Tesamorelin + Ipamorelin + GHK-Cu + PTD-DBM + TB-4

Overview

- Tesamorelin is a GHRH (Growth Hormone Releasing Hormone)

- Ipamorelin is the mildest of GHRPs (Growth Hormone Releasing Peptide)

- GHK-Cu is a naturally occurring copper peptide found in human plasma. As people age, they naturally lose the ability to produce this

- PTD-DBM is a topical man-made peptide to fight hair loss

- Thymosin Beta-4 (TB-4) is related to thymosin, a hormone that is secreted by your thymus, with its main function to produce T cells, which is an essential aspect of the immune system

Why Add These Together?

- Tesamorelin goes up to the anterior pituitary gland and signals the body to create growth hormone (Stronger than MOD-GRF-1-29)

- Ipamorelin works by inhibiting somatostatin on the hypothalamus to allow the release of growth hormone

- GHK-Cu increases collagen, stem cell production, and bone formation by stimulating chondrocytes in bones. GHK-Cu blocks the release of oxidative damage and enhances angiogenesis (development of new blood cells)

- PTD-DBM both prevents hair loss and promotes the growth of new hair follicles by interfering with the CXXC5 protein binding

- Thymosin Beta-4 works by binding to actin, which is a protein that influences the action and formation of most cells in our body.

Enhancing the mechanism of actin, leads to faster healing time, especially in injured areas.

- Thymosin Beta-4 is known to promote hair growth

- Combining these peptides ensures the creation and release of growth hormone occurs simultaneously while adding multiple anti-aging and cosmetic enhancing benefits, especially in regards to hair growth

Research Benefits

Benefits

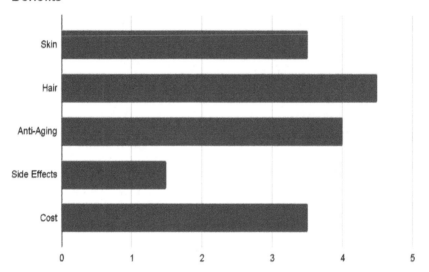

- Increase in the creation and release of endogenous growth hormone

- Promotes muscle growth

- Helps with mood and stress resilience

- Slows down aging

- Improves sleep

- Tightens loose skin and enhances skin elasticity

- Promotes hair growth

- Improves bone density

Research Side Effects

- Redness, itchiness, and swelling of injection sites

- Water retention

- Facial flushing

- Possibility for copper toxicity

- Temporarily tired

- A sharp increase in IGF-1 levels

Matthew's Personal Insight on Research Dosing

- TB-4

  - ¤ 300-1000 mcg per injection

- Tesamorelin

  - ¤ 500-2000 mcg per injection

- Ipamorelin

  - ¤ 100-300 mcg per injection

- GHK-Cu

  - ¤ For subcutaneous injections: 1-2 mg per day

  - ¤ For topical: apply to the area of healing

- PTD-DBM

  - ¤ PTD-DBM sprays are usually available as a 0.001% solution in 25 ml of spray bottles

Matthew's Personal Insight on Research Cycling

- Tesamorelin, Ipamorelin

  - ¤ Multiple injections can be given a day to increase GH secretion. Often used in bodybuilding

  - ¤ 5 days on, 2 days off, 10-12 weeks on, 4-8 weeks off

  - ¤ Carbohydrates and fatty acids can blunt growth hormone release. Best taken 30 minutes before eating or 2 hours after eating

- GHK-Cu

  - ¤ For subcutaneous injection

  - ¤ 6-week intervals

  - ¤ Can be cycled 3-4x a year

- For topical use

  - ¤ Continual use

- PTD-DBM

  - ¤ Use topical spray 1-2 a week

- TB-4

  - ¤ 3-5x a week, 10-12 weeks on, 4-8 weeks off

Matthew's Personal Insight on Timing & Benefits - For Ipamorelin/Tesamorelin

- Burning Fat

  - ¤ Before a workout in a fasted state

- Building Muscle

- ¤ After a workout in a fasted state
- Sleep
  - ¤ Before bed in a fasted state
- General Anti-Aging
  - ¤ In the morning in a fasted state

Matthew's Personal Insight on Timing & Benefits - For GHK-Cu/PTD-DBM

- For Skin
  - ¤ Best to apply after micro-needling
- For Hair
  - ¤ Best to apply after a shower. This will prevent the hair's natural oil from stopping PTD-DBM and GHK-Cu to be absorbed
  - ¤ Absorption and hair growth can be enhanced by micro-needling before applying
  - ¤ Valproic acid is recommended to apply with PTD-DBM for maximal benefits

Matthew's Opinion

- Ipamorelin and Tesamorelin is the gold standard peptide combo for increasing endogenous growth hormone, giving a nice boost in several cosmetic properties
- I have been wanting to try PTD-DBM, as it seems promising and a great peptide to add to a cosmetic stack, especially if hair growth is the focus

- I have never tried TB-4 for hair growth, but it seems promising, and it has several other regenerative benefits

- I would use GHK-Cu topically (skin and hair) and inject to get the most results

- It is important to micro-needle before applying topical GHK-Cu & PTD-DBM to get the most absorption and results

Tesamorelin + Ipamorelin + GHK-Cu + PTD-DBM + TB-4 + BPC-157

Overview

- Tesamorelin is a GHRH (Growth Hormone Releasing Hormone)

- Ipamorelin is the mildest of GHRPs (Growth Hormone Releasing Peptide)

- GHK-Cu is a naturally occurring copper peptide found in human plasma. As people age, they naturally lose the ability to produce this

- PTD-DBM is a topical man-made peptide to fight hair loss

- BPC-157 stands for body-protective compound. It was discovered in the human gastric juice

- Thymosin Beta-4 (TB-4) is related to thymosin, a hormone that is secreted by your thymus, with its main function to produce T cells, which is an essential aspect of the immune system

Why Add These Together?

- Tesamorelin goes up to the anterior pituitary gland and signals the body to create and release growth hormone (Stronger than MOD-GRF-1-29)

- Ipamorelin works by inhibiting somatostatin on the hypothalamus to allow the release of growth hormone

- GHK-Cu increases collagen, stem cell production, and bone formation by stimulating chondrocytes in bones. GHK-Cu blocks the release of oxidative damage and enhances angiogenesis (development of new blood cells)

- PTD-DBM both prevents hair loss and promotes the growth of new hair follicles by interfering with the CXXC5 protein binding

- Thymosin Beta-4 works by binding to actin, which is a protein that influences the action and formation of most cells in our body. Enhancing the mechanism of actin, leads to faster healing time, especially in injured areas

- Thymosin Beta-4 is known to promote hair growth

- BPC-157 is neuroprotective (brain), cardioprotective (heart), gastroprotective (stomach), and musculoskeletal protective (joints, ligaments and muscles)

- BPC-157 enhances growth hormone absorption

- PTD-DBM both prevents hair loss and promotes the growth of new hair follicles by interfering with the CXXC5 protein binding

- Combining these peptides ensures the creation and release of growth hormone occurs simultaneously while adding multiple anti-aging and cosmetic enhancing benefits, especially in regards to hair growth

Research Benefits

Benefits

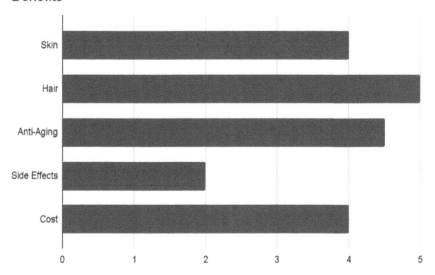

- Increase in the creation and release of endogenous growth hormone

- Promotes muscle growth

- Helps with mood and stress resilience

- Neuroprotective (brain), cardioprotective (heart), gastroprotective (stomach), and musculoskeletal protective (joints, ligaments and muscles)

- Slows down aging

- Improves sleep

- Tightens loose skin and enhances skin elasticity

- Promotes hair growth

- Improves bone density

Research Side Effects

- Redness, itchiness, and swelling of injection sites

- Water retention

- Facial flushing

- Possibility for copper toxicity

- Temporarily tired

- A sharp increase in IGF-1 levels

Matthew's Personal Insight on Research Dosing

- BPC-157

  - 300-600 mcg per injection

- TB-4

  - 300-1000 mcg per injection

- Tesamorelin

  - 500-2000 mcg per injection

- Ipamorelin

  - 100-300 mcg per injection

- GHK-Cu

  - For subcutaneous injections: 1-2 mg per day

  - For topical: apply to the area of healing

- PTD-DBM

  - PTD-DBM sprays are usually available as a 0.001% solution in 25 ml of spray bottles

Matthew's Personal Insight on Research Cycling

- Tesamorelin, Ipamorelin

  - ⌻ Multiple injections can be given a day to increase GH secretion. Often used in bodybuilding

  - ⌻ 5 days on, 2 days off, 10-12 weeks on, 4-8 weeks off

  - ⌻ Carbohydrates and fatty acids can blunt growth hormone release. Best taken 30 minutes before eating or 2 hours after eating

- GHK-Cu

  - ⌻ For subcutaneous injection

  - ⌻ 6-week intervals

  - ⌻ Can be cycled 3-4x a year

- For topical use

  - ⌻ Continual use

- PTD-DBM

  - ⌻ Use topical spray 1-2 a week

- TB-4, BPC-157

  - ⌻ 3-5x a week, 10-12 weeks on, 4-8 weeks off

Matthew's Personal Insight on Research Timing & Benefits - For Ipamorelin/Tesamorelin

- Burning Fat

  - ⌻ Before a workout in a fasted state

- Building Muscle

- ¤ After a workout in a fasted state

- Sleep

  - ¤ Before bed in a fasted state

- General Anti-Aging

  - ¤ In the morning in a fasted state

Matthew's Personal Insight on Research Timing & Benefits - For GHK-Cu/PTD-DBM

- For Skin

  - ¤ Best to apply after micro-needling

- For Hair

  - ¤ Best to apply after a shower. This will prevent the hair's natural oil from stopping PTD-DBM and GHK-Cu to be absorbed

  - ¤ Absorption and hair growth can be enhanced by micro-needling before applying

  - ¤ Valproic acid is recommended to apply with PTD-DBM for maximal benefits

Matthew's Opinion

- Ipamorelin and Tesamorelin is the gold standard peptide combo for increasing endogenous growth hormone, giving a nice boost in several cosmetic properties

- I have been wanting to try PTD-DBM, as it seems promising and a great peptide to add to a cosmetic stack, especially if hair growth is the focus

- I have never tried TB-4 for hair growth, but it seems promising and it has several other regenerative benefits

- I like how BPC-157 enhances the absorption of the growth hormone while adding several anti-aging benefits

- I would use GHK-Cu topically (skin and hair) and inject to get the most results

- It is important to micro-needle before applying topical GHK-Cu & PTD-DBM to get the most absorption and results

15. Peptides Combos for Immunity

TA-1 + TB-4

Overview

- Thymosin Alpha 1 is a peptide that is naturally produced by the thymus gland

- Thymosin Beta-4 (TB-4) is related to thymosin, a hormone that is secreted by your thymus, with its main function to produce T cells, which is an essential aspect of the immune system

Why Add These Together?

- Thymosin Beta-4 works by binding to actin, which is a protein that influences the action and formation of most cells in the body. Enhancing the mechanism of actin leads to faster healing time, especially in injured areas.

- Additionally, binding to actin increases the number of immune system cells and decreases inflammatory substances (cytokine)

- Thymosin alpha 1 strengthens the immune system in numerous ways and addresses both aspects of the immune system (TH1-innate and TH2-acquired) immunity to help return to homeostasis

- Combining these peptides activates and strengthens both aspects of the immune system while having several full-body regenerative benefits

Research Benefits

Benefits

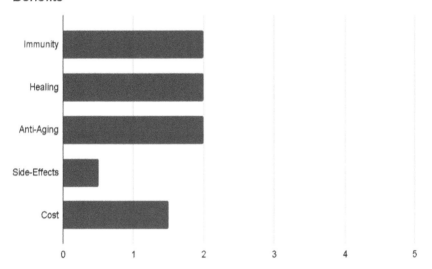

- Eradicates bacteria, viruses, and fungi

- Boosts the function of certain immune cells

- Suppresses cancer and tumor growth

- Accelerates the wound-healing process

- Fights inflammation

- Enhances antibody responses

- Balances TH1/TH2

- Promotes nerve regeneration

Research Side Effects

- Redness, itchiness, and swelling of the injection site

- Feeling temporarily tired

Matthew's Personal Insight on Research Dosing

- TB-4

  ¤ 300 mcg to 1 mg per subcutaneous injection

- TA-1

  ¤ 1-1.5 mg per subcutaneous injection

Matthew's Personal Insight on Research Cycling

- TB-4

  ¤ This can be taken daily for up to 3 months or until the condition resolves

  ¤ Cycle length depends on the health status and response to treatment

  ¤ Take a 1-month break if needed to cycle long-term

- TA-1

  ¤ Every third day

  ¤ 2 weeks to 3 months or longer. The cycle depends on the response and overall health status

Matthew's Opinion

- This would be my go-to peptide stack if I wanted to work on anything immune-related

- Both of these peptides are well-used and well-researched

- I like how both of these peptides offer a wide ray of benefits, especially regarding the immune system with a high safety profile

- I would work closely with a doctor when using these peptides to help determine cycle length and intensity

TA-1 + TB-4 + BPC-157

Overview

- Thymosin Alpha 1 is a peptide that is naturally produced by the thymus gland

- Thymosin Beta-4 (TB-4) is related to thymosin, a hormone that is secreted by your thymus, with its main function to produce T cells, which is an essential aspect of the immune system

- BPC-157 stands for body-protective compound. It was discovered in the human gastric juice

Why Add These Together?

- Thymosin Beta-4 works by binding to actin, which is a protein that influences the action and formation of most cells in the body. Enhancing the mechanism of actin leads to faster healing time, especially in injured areas.

- Additionally, binding to actin increases the number of immune system cells and decreases inflammatory substances (cytokine)

- Thymosin alpha 1 strengthens the immune system in numerous ways and addresses both aspects of the immune system (TH1-innate and TH2-acquired) immunity to help return to homeostasis

- BPC-157 is neuroprotective (brain), cardioprotective (heart), gastroprotective (stomach), and musculoskeletal protective (joints, ligaments and muscles)

- All 3 of these peptides are commonly used together and have a strong synergistic effect

- Combining these peptides activates and strengthens both aspects of the immune system while having several full-body regenerative benefits

Research Benefits

Benefits

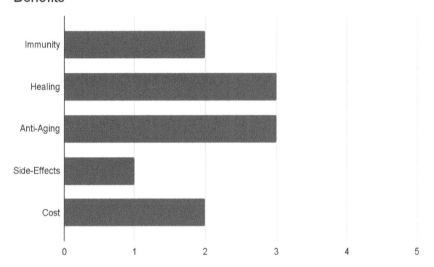

- Eradicates bacteria, viruses, and fungi

- Boosts the function of certain immune cells

- Suppresses cancer and tumor growth

- Accelerates the wound-healing process

- Fights inflammation

- Enhances antibody responses

- Balances TH1/TH2

- Promotes nerve regeneration

- Neuroprotective (brain), cardioprotective (heart), gastroprotective (stomach), and musculoskeletal protective (joints, ligaments and muscles)

Research Side Effects

- Redness, itchiness, and swelling of the injection site

- Feeling temporarily tired

- Water retention

Matthew's Personal Insight on Research Dosing

- TB-4

  ¤ 300 mcg to 1 mg per subcutaneous injection

- TA-1

  ¤ 1-1.5 mg per subcutaneous injection

- BPC-157

  ¤ 400-600 mcg per subcutaneous injection

Matthew's Personal Insight on Research Cycling

- TB-4, BPC-157

  ¤ This can be taken daily for up to 3 months or until the condition resolves

  ¤ Cycle length depends on the health status and response to treatment

  ¤ Take a 1-month break if needed to cycle long-term

- TA-1

  - ¤ Every third day

  - ¤ 2 weeks to 3 months or longer. The cycle depends on the response and overall health status

Matthew's Opinion

- I love all of these peptides since they're all well-used, well-researched, offer a wide ray of benefits, and have a high safety profile

- I would work closely with a doctor when using these peptides to help determine cycle length and intensity.

TA-1 + TB-4 + BPC-157 + KPV

Overview

- Thymosin Alpha 1 is a peptide that is naturally produced by the thymus gland

- Thymosin Beta-4 (TB-4) is related to thymosin, a hormone that is secreted by your thymus, with its main function to produce T cells, which is an essential aspect of the immune system

- BPC-157 stands for body-protective compound. It was discovered in the human gastric juice

- KPV is naturally produce in the body and is found in the hormone alpha-MSH

Why Add These Together?

- Thymosin Beta-4 works by binding to actin, which is a protein that influences the action and formation of most cells in the body. Enhancing the mechanism of actin leads to faster healing time, especially in injured areas.

- Additionally, binding to actin increases the number of immune system cells and decreases inflammatory substances (cytokine)

- Thymosin alpha 1 strengthens the immune system in numerous ways and addresses both aspects of the immune system (TH1-innate and TH2-acquired) immunity to help return to homeostasis

- KPV can enter cells and nuclei, where DNA is. Inside, it can inhibit NF-kB, one of the cell's main controllers of inflammation.

- KPV is most commonly used for autoimmune and inflammatory conditions

- BPC-157 is neuroprotective (brain), cardioprotective (heart), gastroprotective (stomach), and musculoskeletal protective (joints, ligaments and muscles)

- Combining these peptides activates and strengthens both aspects of the immune system while having several full-body regenerative benefits

Research Benefits

Benefits

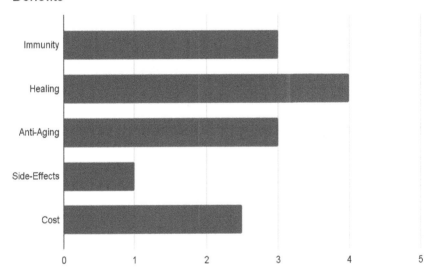

- Eradicates bacteria, viruses, and fungi

- Reduces inflammatory cytokines

- Boosts the function of certain immune cells

- Suppresses cancer and tumor growth

- Accelerates the wound-healing process

- Fights inflammation

- Enhances antibody responses

- Balances TH1/TH2

- Promotes nerve regeneration

- Neuroprotective (brain), cardioprotective (heart), gastroprotective (stomach), and musculoskeletal protective (joints, ligaments and muscles)

Research Side Effects

- Redness, itchiness, and swelling of the injection site

- Feeling temporarily tired

- Water retention

Matthew's Personal Insight on Research Dosing

- TB-4

  ¤ 300 mcg to 1 mg per subcutaneous injection

- TA-1

  ¤ 1-1.5 mg per subcutaneous injection

- BPC-157

  ¤ 400-600 mcg per subcutaneous injection

- KPV

  ¤ Subcutaneous: 200-500 mcg, one time a day

    ◆ Best used for overall inflammation

  ¤ Oral: 250 mcg, twice a day on an empty stomach

- Best used for any stomach/GI inflammation

  ⌑ Topical: 7.5 mg applied 2x a day to area

- Best used for wound healing

Matthew's Personal Insight on Research Cycling

- TB-4, BPC-157, KPV

  ⌑ This can be taken daily for up to 3 months or until the condition resolves

  ⌑ Cycle length depends on the health status and response to treatment

  ⌑ Take a 1-month break if needed to cycle for long-term

- TA-1

  ⌑ Every third day

  ⌑ 2 weeks to 3 months or longer. The cycle depends on the response and overall health status

Matthew's Opinion

- TB-4, TA-1, and BPC-157 are all well-used, well-researched, offer a wide ray of benefits, and have a high safety profile, especially regarding immunity enhancement

- I like how KPV can enter a cell's nucleus and can be taken/applied in various forms

- I would stick with injecting KPV to keep these peptides efficient unless I have an open wound or a specific condition I'm working on

- Combining oral BPC-157 and oral KPV could be a powerful stack to help with any GI issues

- I would work closely with a doctor when using these peptides to help determine cycle length and intensity

TA-1 + TB-4 + BPC-157 + KPV + Humanin

Overview

- Thymosin Alpha 1 is a peptide that is naturally produced by the thymus gland

- Thymosin Beta-4 (TB-4) is related to thymosin, a hormone that is secreted by your thymus, with its main function to produce T cells, which is an essential aspect of the immune system

- BPC-157 stands for body-protective compound. It was discovered in the human gastric juice

- KPV is naturally produce in the body and is found in the hormone alpha-MSH

- Humanin is a peptide found naturally in the mitochondria and many other parts of the human body, such as the heart, kidney, brain, and skeletal muscles.

Why Add These Together?

- Thymosin Beta-4 works by binding to actin, which is a protein that influences the action and formation of most cells in our body. Enhancing the mechanism of actin leads to faster healing time, especially in injured areas.

- Additionally, binding to actin increases the number of immune system cells and decreases inflammatory substances (cytokine)

- Thymosin alpha 1 strengthens the immune system in numerous ways and addresses both aspects of the immune system (TH1-innate and TH2-acquired) immunity to help return to homeostasis

- BPC-157 is neuroprotective (brain), cardioprotective (heart), gastroprotective (stomach), and musculoskeletal protective (joints, ligaments and muscles)

- KPV can enter cells and nuclei, where the DNA is. Inside, it can inhibit NF-kB, one of the cell's main controllers of inflammation.

- KPV is most commonly used for autoimmune and inflammatory conditions

- Humanin plays a role in returning the body to optimal function during a metabolic stress response and has been linked to largely influencing the health span and lifespan

- Combining these peptides activates and strengthens both aspects of the immune system while having several full-body regenerative benefits

Research Benefits

Benefits

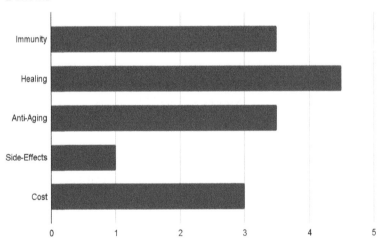

- Eradicates bacteria, viruses, and fungi

- Boosts mitochondria function

384

- Boosts the function of certain immune cells

- Suppresses cancer and tumor growth

- Accelerates the wound-healing process

- Fights inflammation

- Enhances antibody responses

- Balances TH1/TH2

- Promotes nerve regeneration

- Neuroprotective (brain), cardioprotective (heart), gastroprotective (stomach), and musculoskeletal protective (joints, ligaments and muscles)

Research Side Effects

- Redness, itchiness, and swelling of injection site

- Feeling temporarily tired

- Water retention

Matthew's Personal Insight on Research Dosing

- TB-4

  ¤ 300 mcg to 1-gram subcutaneous injection

- TA-1

  ¤ 1-1.5 mg per subcutaneous injection

- BPC-157

  ¤ 400-600 mcg per subcutaneous injection

- Humanin

  - ☐ .04 mg/kg as the therapeutic dose

  - ☐ Weigh 80kg -> 3.2 mg

  - ☐ Weigh 90 kg -> 3.6 mg

  - ☐ Weigh 100 kg -> 4 mg

- KPV

  - ☐ Subcutaneous: 200-500 mcg, one time a day

    - ◆ Best used for overall inflammation

  - ☐ Oral: 250 mcg, twice a day on an empty stomach

    - ◆ Best used for any stomach/GI inflammation

  - ☐ Topical: 7.5 mg applied 2x a day to area

    - ◆ Best used for wound healing

Matthew's Personal Insight on Research Cycling

- TB-4, BPC-157, KPV, Humanin

  - ☐ This can be taken daily for up to 3 months or until the condition resolves

  - ☐ Cycle length depends on the health status and response to treatment

  - ☐ Take a 1-month break if needed to cycle long-term

- TA-1

  - ☐ Every third day

  - ☐ 2 weeks to 3 months or longer. The cycle depends on the response and overall health status

Matthew's Opinion

- TB-4, TA-1, and BPC-157 are all well-used, well-researched, offer a wide ray of benefits, and have a high safety profile, especially regarding immunity enhancement

- I like how KPV can enter a cell's nucleus and can be taken/applied in various forms

- I would stick with injecting KPV to keep stacking these peptides efficient unless I have an open wound or a specific condition I'm working on

- I like how Humanin has been linked to largely influencing the health span and lifespan. It regulates and enhances mitochondrial health, which could be a significant recovery benefit when suffering from anything immune-related

- Combining oral BPC-157 and oral KPV could be a powerful stack to help with any GI issues

- I would work closely with a doctor when using these peptides to help determine cycle length and intensity

TA-1 + TB-4 + BPC-157 + KPV + Humanin + LL-37

Overview

- Thymosin Alpha 1 is a peptide that is naturally produced by the thymus gland

- Thymosin Beta-4 (TB-4) is related to thymosin, a hormone that is secreted by your thymus, with its main function to produce T cells, which is an essential aspect of the immune system

- BPC-157 stands for body-protective compound. It was discovered in the human gastric juice

- KPV is naturally produce in the body and is found in the hormone alpha-MSH

- Humanin is a peptide found naturally in the mitochondria and many other parts of the human body, such as the heart, kidney, brain, and skeletal muscles.

- LL-37 is produced naturally in neutrophils, natural killer cells, and in many different body systems

Why Add These Together?

- Thymosin Beta-4 works by binding to actin, a protein that influences the action and formation of most cells in the body. Enhancing the mechanism of actin leads to faster healing time, especially in injured areas.

- Additionally, binding to actin increases the number of immune system cells and decreases inflammatory substances (cytokine)

- Thymosin alpha 1 strengthens the immune system in numerous ways and addresses both aspects of the immune system (TH1-innate and TH2-acquired) immunity to help return to homeostasis

- LL-37 has the potential to serve as an alternative to antibiotics and plays a vital role in innate and adaptive immunity

- BPC-157 is neuroprotective (brain), cardioprotective (heart), gastroprotective (stomach), and musculoskeletal protective (joints, ligaments and muscles)

- KPV can enter cells and nuclei, where the DNA is. Inside, it can inhibit NF-kB, one of the cell's main controllers of inflammation.

- KPV is most commonly used for autoimmune and inflammatory conditions

- Humanin plays a role in returning the body to optimal function during a metabolic stress response and has been linked to largely influencing the health span and lifespan

- Combining these peptides activates and strengthens both aspects of the immune system while having several full-body regenerative benefits

Research Benefits

Benefits

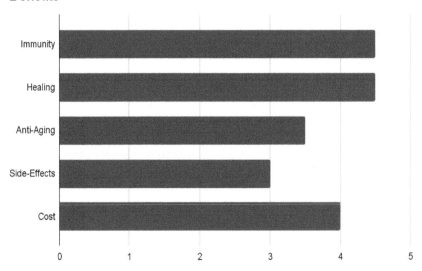

- Eradicates bacteria, viruses, and fungi

- Boosts mitochondria function

- Boosts the function of certain immune cells

- Suppresses cancer and tumor growth

- Accelerates the wound-healing process

- Fights inflammation

- Enhances antibody responses

- Balances TH1/TH2

- Promotes nerve regeneration

- Neuroprotective (brain), cardioprotective (heart), gastroprotective (stomach), and musculoskeletal protective (joints, ligaments and muscles)

Research Side Effects

- Redness, itchiness, and swelling of the injection site

- Feeling temporarily tired

- Water retention

- LL-37

- Induction of autoimmune disease (high LL-37 is found in subjects with autoimmune diseases)

- Damage to sperm surface membranes

- Toxic to both bacterial and normal cells

Matthew's Personal Insight on Research Dosing

- TB-4

  ¤ 300 mcg to 1 mg per subcutaneous injection

- TA-1

  ¤ 1-1.5 mg per subcutaneous injection

- BPC-157

  ¤ 400-600 mcg per subcutaneous injection

- Humanin

  ¤ .04 mg/kg as the therapeutic dose

  ¤ Weigh 80kg -> 3.2 mg

- Weigh 90 kg -> 3.6 mg

- Weigh 100 kg -> 4 mg

• LL-37

- 100 mcg per injection

• KPV

- Subcutaneous: 200-500 mcg, one time a day

  ◆ Best used for overall inflammation

- Oral: 250 mcg, twice a day on an empty stomach

  ◆ Best used for any stomach/GI inflammation

- Topical: 7.5 mg applied 2x a day to area

  ◆ Best used for wound healing

Matthew's Personal Insight on Research Cycling

• LL-37

- It can be given 2x a day. Once in the morning and once at night

- 4–6-week cycle and then evaluate response and status

• TB-4, BPC-157, KPV, Humanin

- This can be taken daily for up to 3 months or until the condition resolves

- Cycle length depends on the health status and response to treatment

- Take a 1-month break if needed to cycle for long-term

- TA-1

    - ¤ Every third day

    - ¤ 2 weeks to 3 months or longer. The cycle depends on the response and overall health status

Matthew's Opinion

- TB-4, TA-1, and BPC-157 are all well-used, well-researched, offer a wide ray of benefits, and have a high safety profile, especially regarding immunity enhancement

- I like how KPV can enter a cell's nucleus and can be taken/applied in various forms

- I would stick with injecting KPV to keep stacking these peptides efficient unless I have an open wound or a specific condition I'm working on

- I like how Humanin has been linked to largely influencing the health span and lifespan. It regulates and enhances mitochondrial health, which could be a major recovery benefit when suffering from anything immune-related

- Combining oral BPC-157 and oral KPV could be a powerful stack to help with any GI issues

- LL-37 is a potent immune peptide that I would only use if I worked closely with a doctor. The risk of damaging my body and causing the opposite effect makes it risky

- I would work closely with a doctor when using these peptides to help determine cycle length and intensity

TA-1 + TB-4 + BPC-157 + KPV + Humanin + LL-37 + ARA-290/VIP

Overview

- Thymosin Alpha 1 is a peptide that is naturally produced by the thymus gland

- Thymosin Beta-4 (TB-4) is related to thymosin, a hormone that is secreted by your thymus, with its main function to produce T cells, which is an essential aspect of the immune system

- BPC-157 stands for body-protective compound. It was discovered in the human gastric juice

- KPV is naturally produce in the body and is found in the hormone alpha-MSH

- Humanin is a peptide found naturally in the mitochondria and many other parts of the human body, such as the heart, kidney, brain, and skeletal muscles.

- LL-37 is produced naturally in neutrophils, natural killer cells, and in many different body systems

- Vasoactive Intestinal Peptide (VIP) is a neuropeptide naturally found in the intestines, pancreas, brain, central nervous system, urogenital system, lungs, and all over the body

- ARA-290 is a peptide designed off a segment of the hormone erythropoietin

Why Add These Together?

- Thymosin Beta-4 works by binding to actin, a protein that influences the action and formation of most cells in the body. Enhancing the mechanism of actin leads to faster healing time, especially in injured areas.

- Additionally, binding to actin increases the number of immune system cells and decreases inflammatory substances (cytokine)

- Thymosin alpha 1 strengthens the immune system in numerous ways and addresses both aspects of the immune system (TH1-innate and TH2-acquired) immunity to help return to homeostasis

- LL-37 has the potential to serve as an alternative to antibiotics and plays an important role in innate and adaptive immunity

- BPC-157 is neuroprotective (brain), cardioprotective (heart), gastroprotective (stomach), and musculoskeletal protective (joints, ligaments and muscles)

- KPV can enter cells and nuclei, where the DNA is. Inside, it can inhibit NF-kB, one of the cell's main controllers of inflammation.

- KPV is most commonly used for autoimmune and inflammatory conditions

- Humanin plays a role in returning the body to optimal function during a metabolic stress response and has been linked to largely influencing the health span and lifespan

- VIP is a great to help aid in blood circulation and blood pressure control

- ARA-290 is excellent for helping with diabetes or neuropathy

- Combining these peptides activates and strengthens both aspects of the immune system while having several full-body regenerative benefits, with additional support for either diabetes or blood circulation

Research Benefits

Benefits

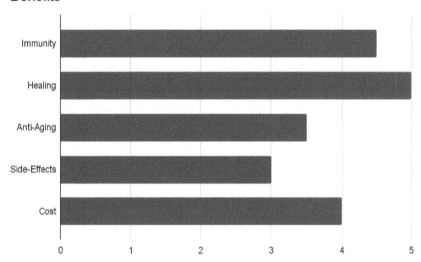

- Eradicates bacteria, viruses, and fungi

- Boosts mitochondria function

- Regulates blood pressure

- Fights diabetes

- Boosts the function of certain immune cells

- Suppresses cancer and tumor growth

- Accelerates the wound-healing process

- Fights inflammation

- Enhances antibody responses

- Balances TH1/TH2

- Promotes nerve regeneration

- Neuroprotective (brain), cardioprotective (heart), gastroprotective (stomach), and musculoskeletal protective (joints, ligaments and muscles)

Research Side Effects

- Redness, itchiness, and swelling of the injection site

- Feeling temporarily tired

- Water retention

- Low blood pressure (VIP)

- LL-37

  ¤ Induction of autoimmune disease (high LL-37 is found in subjects with autoimmune diseases)

  ¤ Damage to sperm surface membranes

  ¤ Toxic to both bacterial and normal cells

Matthew's Personal Insight on Research Dosing

- TB-4

  ¤ 300 mcg to 1 mg per subcutaneous injection

- TA-1

  ¤ 1-1.5 mg per subcutaneous injection

- BPC-157

  ¤ 400-600 mcg per subcutaneous injection

- Humanin

  - ¤ .04 mg/kg as the therapeutic dose

  - ¤ Weigh 80kg -> 3.2 mg

  - ¤ Weigh 90 kg -> 3.6 mg

  - ¤ Weigh 100 kg -> 4 mg

- ARA-290

  - ¤ 4mg/day through a subcutaneous injection

- VIP

  - ¤ 50 mcg sprayed in each nostril

- LL-37

  - ¤ 100 mcg per injection

- KPV

  - ¤ Subcutaneous: 200-500 mcg, one time a day

    - ◆ Best used for overall inflammation

  - ¤ Oral: 250 mcg, twice a day on an empty stomach

    - ◆ Best used for any stomach/GI inflammation

  - ¤ Topical: 7.5 mg applied 2x a day to area

    - ◆ Best used for wound healing

Matthew's Personal Insight on Research Cycling

- LL-37

  - ¤ It can be given 2x a day. Once in the morning and once at night

  - ¤ 4–6-week cycle and then evaluate response and status

- TB-4, BPC-157, KPV, Humanin, ARA-290

  - ¤ This can be taken daily for up to 3 months or until the condition resolves

  - ¤ Cycle length depends on the health status and response to treatment

  - ¤ Take a 1-month break if needed to cycle for long-term

- TA-1

  - ¤ Every third day

  - ¤ 2 weeks to 3 months or longer. The cycle depends on the response and overall health status

- VIP

  - ¤ 1-16 times a day

  - ¤ This peptide is fast-acting with a short half-life (2 minutes)

  - ¤ It is best to use this peptide when an enhanced blood flow or muscle relaxation in an area is needed

  - ¤ Frequency and intensity depends on the response and condition

  - ¤ The goal is not to become dependent on the compound

Matthew's Opinion

- TB-4, TA-1, and BPC-157 are all well-used, well-researched, offer a wide ray of benefits, and have a high safety profile, especially regarding immunity enhancement

- I like how KPV can enter a cell's nucleus and can be taken/applied in various forms

- I would stick with injecting KPV to keep stacking these peptides efficient unless I have an open wound or a specific condition I'm working on

- I like how Humanin has been linked to largely influencing the health span and lifespan. It regulates and enhances mitochondrial health, which could be a major recovery benefit when suffering from anything immune-related

- Combining oral BPC-157 and oral KPV could be a powerful stack to help with any GI issues

- Depending on the conditions, I would pick between ARA-290 and VIP. Both of these peptides target the symptoms rather than the root cause

- VIP is great for blood circulation and blood pressure control

- ARA-290 is great for diabetics

- LL-37 is a powerful immune peptide that I would only use if I worked closely with a doctor. The risk of damaging my body and causing the opposite effect makes it risky

- I would work closely with a doctor when using these peptides to help determine cycle length and intensity

16. Peptides Combos for Sexual Health

Kisspeptin-10 + PT-141

Overview

- Kisspeptin-10 is a neuropeptide hormone from the hypothalamus and is often called the "puberty" peptide

- PT-141 is a libido-boosting peptide targeting the melanocortin receptors (MC3R and MC4R)

Why Add These Together?

- PT-141 works on the MC4R and MC3R receptors in the hypothalamus, which signals receptors in the central nervous system to enhance blood flow, libido, and arousal

- Kisspeptin-10 allows for the release of LH (Luteinizing Hormone) and FSH (Follicle Stimulating Hormone) in the pituitary

- In men, LH and FSH signal the testes to create more testosterone and sperm

- In women, LH & FSH signals the ovaries to make more estrogen and signals the release of an egg (ovulation)

- Combining these peptides enhances sex hormones and fertility with a fast-acting increase in blood flow, libido, and arousal

Research Benefits

Benefits

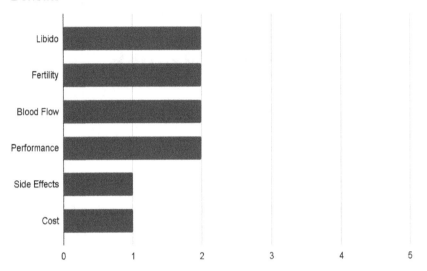

- Increases sexual desire, motivation, and arousal across genders

- Induces erectile response

- Improves genital sensation and pleasure

- May help with discomfort and orgasm during intercourse

- May help with emotional issues around sex

- Increases sex hormones in both males and females (testosterone, estrogen)

- Enhances fertility

- Temporarily increases oxytocin

Research Side Effects

- Redness, itchiness, and swelling of injection sites

- Nausea

- Flushing

- Do not use with other PDE-5 inhibitors (Sildenafil, Vardenafil, Tadalafil, Avanafil)

- Use with other PDE-5 can lead to priapism (too long and painful erection)

Matthew's Personal Insight on Research Dosing & Cycling

- Kisspeptin-10

  - 1 mcg per kg

  - Peak FSH & LH occurs 45-60 minutes after injection

  - 3-5x week, 1 month on, 1 month off

- PT-141

  - Typical dosage is around 1 mg but can be increased up to 4 mg

  - One dose per 24 hours at the most. More can lead to desensitization of receptors

  - Effects can last up to 24-72 hours

Matthew's Personal Insight on Research Timing & Benefits

- PT-141

  ¤ Best taken 30-60 minutes before intercourse

- Kisspeptin-10

  ¤ Testosterone Production (Men)

    ◆ Best taken in the morning in a fasted state

  ¤ Fertility

    ◆ Women -> Best taken around ovulation and 45-60 minutes before attempting conception

    ◆ Men -> Best taken around 45-60 minutes before attempting conception

Matthew's Opinion

- I like how PT-141 works on the nervous system and can be used with both men and women.

- I would use it 1-2x week since the effects can last up to 72 hours

- I like how Kisspeptin-10 increases sex hormones with added fertility for male and female

- This is a great beginner stack if sexual health is the primary goal

PT-141 + Kisspeptin-10 + VIP

Overview

- Kisspeptin-10 is a neuropeptide hormone from the hypothalamus and is often called the "puberty" peptide

- PT-141 is a libido-boosting peptide targeting the melanocortin receptors (MC3R and MC4R)

- Vasoactive Intestinal Peptide (VIP) is a neuropeptide naturally found in the intestines, pancreas, brain, central nervous system, urogenital system, lungs, and all over the body

Why Add These Together?

- VIP's main benefit is being a vasodilator, which enhances blood flow. This can help enhance blood flow to penile tissue, helping with erectile dysfunction (ED)

- PT-141 works on the MC4R and MC3R receptors in the hypothalamus, which signals receptors in the central nervous system to enhance blood flow, libido, and arousal

- Kisspeptin-10 allows for the release of LH (Luteinizing Hormone) and FSH (Follicle Stimulating Hormone) in the pituitary

- In men, LH and FSH signal the testes to create more testosterone and sperm

- In women, LH & FSH signals the ovaries to make more estrogen and signals the release of an egg (ovulation)

- Combining these peptides enhances sex hormones, and fertility with a fast-acting increase in blood flow, libido, and arousal

Research Benefits

Benefits

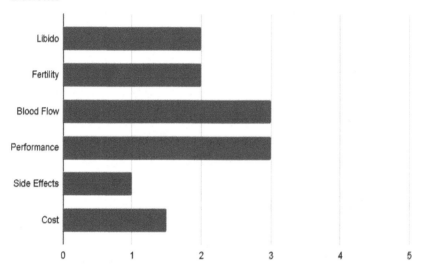

- Increases sexual desire, motivation, and arousal across genders

- Induces erectile response

- Improves genital sensation and pleasure

- May help with discomfort and orgasm during intercourse

- May help with emotional issues around sex

- Increases sex hormones in both males and females (testosterone, estrogen)

- Enhances fertility

- Temporarily increases oxytocin

- Enhances blood flow

Research Side Effects

- Redness, itchiness, and swelling of injection sites

- Nausea

- Flushing

- Low blood pressure

- Do not use with other PDE-5 inhibitors (Sildenafil, Vardenafil, Tadalafil, Avanafil)

- Use with other PDE-5 can lead to priapism (too long and painful erection)

Matthew's Personal Insight on Research Dosing

- VIP

  - ¤ 50 mcg sprayed in each nostril

- Kisspeptin-10

  - ¤ 1 mcg per kg (100-200 mcg)

  - ¤ Peak FSH & LH occurs 45-60 minutes after injection

- PT-141

  - ¤ Typical dosage is around 1 mg but can be increased up to 4 mg

Matthew's Personal Insight on Research Cycling

- VIP

  - ¤ 1-16 times a day

  - ¤ This peptide is fast-acting with a short half-life (2 minutes)

- ¤ Dosing frequency and intensity depends on response and condition

- Kisspeptin-10

  - ¤ 3-5x week, 1 month on, 1 month off

- PT-141

  - ¤ One dose per 24 hours at the most. More can lead to desensitization of receptors

  - ¤ Effects can last up to 24-72 hours

Matthew's Personal Insight on Research Timing & Benefits

- VIP

  - ¤ It is best to use this peptide when the goal is to increase blood flow (Minutes before intercourse)

  - ¤ It could be used during intercourse

- PT-141

  - ¤ Best taken 30-60 minutes before intercourse

- Kisspeptin-10

  - ¤ Testosterone Production (Men)

    - ◆ Best taken in the morning in a fasted state

  - ¤ Fertility

    - ◆ Women -> Best taken around ovulation and 45-60 minutes before attempting conception

- Men -> Best taken around 45-60 minutes before attempting conception

Matthew's Opinion

- VIP is a great addition as it's a fast-acting vasodilator (increases blood flow). It could be useful right before intercourse or during to keep blood flow strong throughout intercourse

- I like how PT-141 works on the nervous system and can be used with both a man and a woman

- I would use it 1-2x week since the effects can last up to 72 hours

- I like how Kisspeptin-10 increases sex hormones with added fertility for male and female

- It is important not to get dependent on PT-141 or VIP. Rather, use it as a way to spice up a sex life every now & then

PT-141 + Kisspeptin-10 + VIP + MOD-GRF-1-29 + Ipamorelin

Overview

- Kisspeptin-10 is a neuropeptide hormone from the hypothalamus and is often called the "puberty" peptide

- PT-141 is a libido-boosting peptide targeting the melanocortin receptors (MC3R and MC4R)

- Vasoactive Intestinal Peptide (VIP) is a neuropeptide naturally found in the intestines, pancreas, brain, central nervous system, urogenital system, lungs, and all over the body

- MOD-GRF-1-29 is a GHRH (Growth Hormone Releasing Hormone)

- Ipamorelin is the mildest of GHRPs (Growth Hormone Releasing Peptide)

Why Add These Together?

- VIP's main benefit is being a vasodilator, which enhances blood flow. This can help enhance blood flow to penile tissue, helping with erectile dysfunction (ED)

- PT-141 works on the MC4R and MC3R receptors in the hypothalamus, which signals receptors in the central nervous system to enhance blood flow, libido, and arousal

- Kisspeptin-10 allows for the release of LH (Luteinizing Hormone) and FSH (Follicle Stimulating Hormone) in the pituitary

- In men, LH and FSH signal the testes to create more testosterone and sperm

410

- In women, LH & FSH signals the ovaries to make more estrogen and signals the release of an egg (ovulation)

- MOD-GRF-1-29 goes up to the anterior pituitary gland and signals the body to create growth hormone

- Ipamorelin works by inhibiting somatostatin on the hypothalamus to allow the release of growth hormone

- Combining these peptides ensures the creation and release of growth hormone occurs simultaneously, enhances sex hormones and fertility with a fast-acting increase in blood flow, libido, and arousal

Research Benefits

Benefits

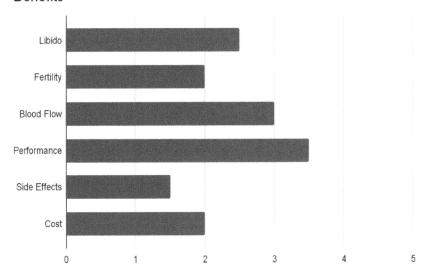

- Increases sexual desire, motivation, and arousal across genders

- Induces erectile response

- Improves genital sensation and pleasure

- May help with discomfort and orgasm during intercourse

- May help with emotional issues around sex

- Increases sex hormones in both males and females (testosterone, estrogen)

- Enhances fertility

- Temporarily increases oxytocin

- Enhances blood flow

- Increase in the creation and release of endogenous growth hormone

Research Side Effects

- Redness, itchiness, and swelling of injection sites

- Nausea

- Flushing

- Low blood pressure

- Water retention

- Facial flushing

- Do not use with other PDE-5 inhibitors (Sildenafil, Vardenafil, Tadalafil, Avanafil)

- Use with other PDE-5 can lead to priapism (too long and painful erection)

Matthew's Personal Insight on Research Dosing

- MOD-GRF-1-29

  ¤ 100 mcg per injection (more is not better)

- Ipamorelin
  - 100-300 mcg per injection
- VIP
  - 50 mcg sprayed in each nostril
- Kisspeptin-10
  - 1 mcg per kg (100-200 mcg)
  - Peak FSH & LH occurs 45-60 minutes after injection
- PT-141
  - Typical dosage is around 1 mg but can be increased up to 4 mg

Matthew's Personal Insight on Research Cycling

- Ipamorelin, MOD-GRF-1-29
  - Multiple injections can be given a day to increase GH secretion. Often used in bodybuilding
  - 5 days on, 2 days off, 10-12 weeks on, 4-8 weeks off
  - Carbohydrates and fatty acids can blunt growth hormone release. Best taken 30 minutes before eating or 2 hours after eating
- Kisspeptin-10
  - 3-5x week, 1 month on, 1 month off
- VIP
  - 1-16 times a day
  - This peptide is fast-acting with a short half-life (2 minutes)
  - Dosing frequency and intensity depends on the response and condition

- PT-141

  - ¤ One dose per 24 hours at the most. More can lead to desensitization of receptors

  - ¤ Effects can last up to 24-72 hours

Matthew's Personal Insight on Research Timing & Benefits

- VIP

  - ¤ It is best to use this peptide when an increase in blood flow is wanted (minutes before intercourse)

  - ¤ It could be used during intercourse

- Kisspeptin-10

  - ¤ Testosterone Production (Men)

    - ◆ Best taken in the morning in a fasted state

  - ¤ Fertility

    - ◆ Women -> Best taken around ovulation and 45-60 minutes before attempting conception

    - ◆ Men -> Best taken around 45-60 minutes before attempting conception

- Ipamorelin, MOD-GRF-1-29

  - ¤ Sexual performance

    - ◆ 30 minutes before intercourse in a fasted state

  - ¤ General performance/anti-aging

    - ◆ Fasted state in the morning

- PT-141

  ⌑ Best taken 30-60 minutes before intercourse

Matthew's Opinion

- MOD-GRF-1-29 and Ipamorelin are my favorite combos for increasing endogenous growth hormone. I believe that having higher levels of growth hormone will indirectly/directly lead to better sexual performance, libido, and arousal since growth hormone heals and enhances numerous aspects of the body

- VIP is a great addition as it's a fast-acting vasodilator (increases blood flow). It could be useful right before intercourse or darning to keep blood flow strong throughout intercourse

- I like how PT-141 works on the nervous system and can be used with both a man and a woman

- I would use it 1-2x week since the effects can last up to 72 hours

- I like how Kisspeptin-10 increases sex hormones with added fertility for male and female

- It is important not to get dependent on PT-141 or VIP. Rather, use it as a way to spice up a sex life every now & then

PT-141 + Kisspeptin-10 + VIP + Tesamorelin + Ipamorelin

Overview

- Kisspeptin-10 is a neuropeptide hormone from the hypothalamus and is often called the "puberty" peptide

- PT-141 is a libido-boosting peptide targeting the melanocortin receptors (MC3R and MC4R)

- Vasoactive Intestinal Peptide (VIP) is a neuropeptide naturally found in the intestines, pancreas, brain, central nervous system, urogenital system, lungs, and all over the body

- Tesamorelin is a GHRH (Growth Hormone Releasing Hormone)

- Pamorelin is the mildest f GHRPs (Growth Harmon)

Why Add These Together?

- VIP's main benefit is being a vasodilator, which enhances blood flow. This can help enhance blood flow to penile tissue, helping with erectile dysfunction (ED)

- PT-141 works on the MC4R and MC3R receptors in the hypothalamus, which signals receptors in the central nervous system to enhance blood flow, libido, and arousal

- Kisspeptin-10 allows for the release of LH (Luteinizing Hormone) and FSH (Follicle Stimulating Hormone) in the pituitary

- In men, LH and FSH signal the testes to create more testosterone and sperm

- In women, LH & FSH signals the ovaries to make more estrogen and signals the release of an egg (ovulation)

416

- Tesamorelin goes up to the anterior pituitary gland and signals the body to create growth hormone (Stronger than MOD-GRF-1-29)

- Ipamorelin works by inhibiting somatostatin on the hypothalamus to allow the release of growth hormone

- Combining these peptides ensures the creation and release of growth hormone occurs simultaneously, enhances sex hormones and fertility with a fast-acting increase in blood flow, libido, and arousal

Research Benefits

Benefits

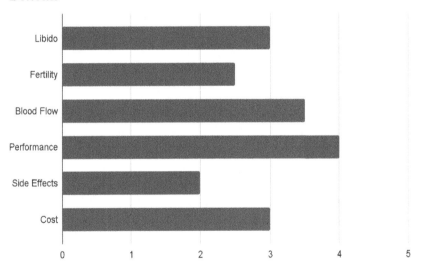

- Increases sexual desire, motivation, and arousal across genders

- Induces erectile response

- Improves genital sensation and pleasure

- May help with discomfort and orgasm during intercourse

- May help with emotional issues around sex

417

- Increases sex hormones in both males and females (testosterone, estrogen)

- Enhances fertility

- Temporarily increases oxytocin

- Enhances blood flow

- Increase in the creation and release of endogenous growth hormone

Research Side Effects

- Redness, itchiness, and swelling of injection sites

- Nausea

- Flushing

- Low blood pressure

- Water retention

- A sharp increase in IGF-1 levels

- Facial flushing

- Do not use with other PDE-5 inhibitors (Sildenafil, Vardenafil, Tadalafil, Avanafil)

- Use with other PDE-5 can lead to priapism (too long and painful erection)

Matthew's Personal Insight on Research Dosing

- Tesamorelin

    ¤ 500-2000 mcg per injection

- Ipamorelin

- ¤ 100-300 mcg per injection

- VIP

  - ¤ 50 mcg sprayed in each nostril

- Kisspeptin-10

  - ¤ 1 mcg per kg (100-200 mcg)

  - ¤ Peak FSH & LH occurs 45-60 minutes after injection

- PT-141

  - ¤ Typical dosage is around 1 mg but can be increased up to 4 mg

Matthew's Personal Insight on Research Cycling

- Ipamorelin, Tesamorelin

  - ¤ Multiple injections can be given a day to increase GH secretion. Often used in bodybuilding

  - ¤ 5 days on, 2 days off, 10-12 weeks on, 4-8 weeks off

  - ¤ Carbohydrates and fatty acids can blunt growth hormone release. Best taken 30 minutes before eating or 2 hours after eating

- Kisspeptin-10

  - ¤ 3-5x week, 1 month on, 1 month off

- VIP

  - ¤ 1-16 times a day

  - ¤ This peptide is fast-acting with a short half-life (2 minutes)

  - ¤ Dosing frequency and intensity depend on the response and condition

- PT-141

  - ¤ One dose per 24 hours at the most. More can lead to desensitization of receptors

  - ¤ Effects can last up to 24-72 hours

Matthew's Personal Insight on Research Timing & Benefits

- VIP

  - ¤ It is best to use this peptide an increase in blood flow is desired (minutes before intercourse)

  - ¤ It could be used during intercourse

- Kisspeptin-10

  - ¤ Testosterone Production (Men)

    - ◆ Best taken in the morning in a fasted state

  - ¤ Fertility

    - ◆ Women -> Best taken around ovulation and 45-60 minutes before attempting conception

    - ◆ Men -> Best taken around 45-60 minutes before attempting conception

- Ipamorelin, Tesamorelin

  - ¤ Sexual performance

    - ◆ 30 minutes before intercourse in a fasted state

  - ¤ General performance/anti-aging

    - ◆ Fasted state in the morning

- PT-141

  ¤ Best taken 30-60 minutes before intercourse

Matthew's Opinion

- Tesamorelin is a nice upgrade replacement from MOD-GRF-1-29. I would start at the lower dosing scheme and work up as I get more comfortable

- Tesamorelin and Ipamorelin are a powerful combo for increasing endogenous growth hormone. I believe that having higher levels of growth hormone will indirectly/directly lead to better sexual performance, libido, and arousal since growth hormone heals and enhances numerous aspects of the body

- I like how PT-141 works on the nervous system and can be used with both a man and a woman

- I would use it 1-2x week since the effects can last up to 72 hours

- I like how Kisspeptin-10 increases sex hormones with added fertility for male and female

- VIP is a great addition as it's a fast-acting vasodilator (increases blood flow). It could be useful right before intercourse or during to keep blood flow strong throughout intercourse

- It is essential not to get dependent on PT-141 or VIP. Instead, use it as a way to spice up a sex life every now & then.

PT-141 + Kisspeptin-10 + VIP + Tesamorelin + Ipamorelin + Melanotan II

Overview

- Kisspeptin-10 is a neuropeptide hormone from the hypothalamus and is often called the "puberty" peptide

- PT-141 is a libido-boosting peptide targeting the melanocortin receptors (MC3R and MC4R)

- Vasoactive Intestinal Peptide (VIP) is a neuropeptide naturally found in the intestines, pancreas, brain, central nervous system, urogenital system, lungs, and all over the body

- Tesamorelin is a GHRH (Growth Hormone Releasing Hormone)

- Ipamorelin is the mildest of GHRPs (Growth Hormone Releasing Peptide)

- Melanotan II works on the melanocortin system and replicates the hormone melanocortin, which is naturally released by the pituitary gland

Why Add These Together?

- VIP's main benefit is being a vasodilator, which enhances blood flow. This can help enhance blood flow to penile tissue, helping with erectile dysfunction (ED)

- PT-141 works on the MC4R and MC3R receptors in the hypothalamus, which signals receptors in the central nervous system to enhance blood flow, libido, and arousal

- Kisspeptin-10 allows for the release of LH (Luteinizing Hormone) and FSH (Follicle Stimulating Hormone) in the pituitary

- In men, LH and FSH signal the testes to create more testosterone and sperm

- In women, LH & FSH signals the ovaries to make more estrogen and signals the release of an egg (ovulation)

- Tesamorelin goes up to the anterior pituitary gland and signals the body to create growth hormone (Stronger than MOD-GRF-1-29)

- Ipamorelin works by inhibiting somatostatin on the hypothalamus to allow the release of growth hormone

- Melanotan II mostly binds to MC1R, MC3R and MC4R receptors

- MC1R (melanogenesis -> tanning)

- MC3R (suppression of appetite)

- MC4R (enhanced sexual stimulus)

- Combining these peptides ensures the creation and release of growth hormone occurs simultaneously, enhances sex hormones and fertility with a fast-acting increase in blood flow, libido, arousal, and a long-acting increase in libido (only for men from Melanotan II)

Research Benefits

Benefits

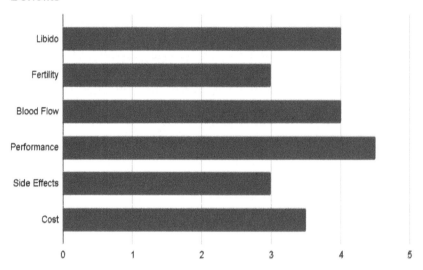

- Increases sexual desire, motivation, and arousal across genders

- Induces erectile response

- Improves genital sensation and pleasure

- May help with discomfort and orgasm during intercourse

- May help with emotional issues around sex

- Increases sex hormones in both males and females (testosterone, estrogen)

- Enhances fertility

- Temporarily increases oxytocin

- Enhances blood flow

- Increase the creation and release of endogenous growth hormone

Research Side Effects

- Redness, itchiness, and swelling of injection sites

- Nausea

- Flushing

- Low blood pressure

- Water retention

- A sharp increase in IGF-1 levels

- Facial flushing

- Do not use Melanotan II if there is history of skin cancer.

- Do not use with other PDE-5 inhibitors (Sildenafil, Vardenafil, Tadalafil, Avanafil)

- Use with other PDE-5 can lead to priapism (too long and painful erection)

Matthew's Personal Insight on Research Dosing

- Melanotan II

  - 200-1000 mcg per injection (fast acting)

  - 100-200 mcg per injection consistently (slow-acting)

- Tesamorelin

  - 500-2000 mcg per injection

- Ipamorelin

  - 100-300 mcg per injection

- VIP

  - ¤ 50 mcg sprayed in each nostril

- Kisspeptin-10

  - ¤ 1 mcg per kg (100-200 mcg)

  - ¤ Peak FSH & LH occurs 45-60 minutes after injection

- PT-141

  - ¤ The typical dosage is around 1 mg but can be increased up to 4 mg

Matthew's Personal Insight on Research Cycling

- Melanotan II

  - ¤ 200-1000 mcg (fast acting) - Dosing frequency and intensity depend on the response and condition. It could be used 30-60 minutes before intercourse

  - ¤ 100-200 mcg (slow acting) - Can be taken daily. It is important to pay close attention to skin tone since Melanotan II darkens skins

- Ipamorelin, Tesamorelin

  - ¤ Multiple injections can be given a day to increase GH secretion. Often used in bodybuilding

  - ¤ 5 days on, 2 days off, 10-12 weeks on, 4-8 weeks off

  - ¤ Carbohydrates and fatty acids can blunt growth hormone release. Best taken 30 minutes before eating or 2 hours after eating

- Kisspeptin-10

  - ¤ 3-5x week, 1 month on, 1 month off

- VIP

  - ¤ 1-16 times a day

  - ¤ This peptide is fast-acting with a short half-life (2 minutes)

  - ¤ Dosing frequency and intensity depends on the response and condition

- PT-141

  - ¤ One dose per 24 hours at the most. More can lead to desensitization of receptors

  - ¤ Effects can last up to 24-72 hours

Matthew's Personal Insight on Research Timing & Benefits

- VIP

  - ¤ It is best to use this peptide when an increase in blood flow is desired (Minutes before intercourse)

  - ¤ It could be used during intercourse

- Kisspeptin-10

  - ¤ Testosterone Production (Men)

    - ◆ Best taken in the morning in a fasted state

  - ¤ Fertility

    - ◆ Women -> Best taken around ovulation and 45-60 minutes before attempting conception

    - ◆ Men -> Best taken around 45-60 minutes before attempting conception

- Melanotan II

  ¤ Best taken 30-60 minutes before intercourse

- Ipamorelin, Tesamorelin

  ¤ Sexual performance

    ◆ 30 minutes before intercourse in a fasted state

  ¤ General performance/anti-aging

    ◆ Fasted state in the morning

- PT-141

  ¤ Best taken 30-60 minutes before intercourse

Matthew's Opinion

- Tesamorelin is a nice upgrade replacement from MOD-GRF-1-29. I would start at the lower dosing scheme and work up as I felt more comfortable

- Tesamorelin and Ipamorelin is a powerful combo for increasing endogenous growth hormone. I believe that having higher levels of growth hormone will indirectly/directly lead to better sexual performance, libido, and arousal since growth hormone heals and enhances numerous aspects of the body

- VIP is a great addition as it's a fast-acting vasodilator (increases blood flow). It could be useful right before intercourse or darning to keep blood flow strong throughout intercourse

- I like how PT-141 works on the nervous system and can be used with both a man and a woman

- I would use it 1-2x week since the effects can last up to 72 hours

- I like how Melanotan II sexual stimulus is gradual over time with longer lasting effects but also can be used in a fast-acting way by increasing the dose

- It is important to be well-educated on Melanotan II since it is a powerful peptide with potential side-effects

- I would use the slow-acting dosing (200 mcg, 2-4x a week) of Melanotan II as this would gradually increase my libido over time, and then use PT-141 and VIP for my fast-acting sexual stimulus

- Combining the fast-acting dosing scheme of Melanotan II (200-1000 mcg) with VIP and PT-141 seems to be too intense and may lead to painful and too-long erections. And, because PT-141 and Melanotan II have a cross-over since they work on similar receptors

- I like how Kisspeptin-10 increases sex hormones with added fertility for male and female

- It is important not to get dependent on PT-141 or VIP. Instead, use it as a way to spice up a sex life every now & then

17. Starting A Peptide Research Lab

Disclaimer

This is how I currently approach all my peptide research. Except for the foregoing disclaimers, when referring to "you," I am referring to myself, as this is how I created the notes for my research techniques. Matthew Farrahi is not a doctor or qualified/accredited healthcare professional and does not promote, recommend, or encourage the use of research compounds for human use, whether directly or indirectly. Research compounds are not for human or animal consumption under any circumstance, in any form, or under any condition. The information displayed in this chapter is strictly for research and informational purposes and is neither intended to be medical advice/opinion nor should be considered as such. Matthew Farrahi is a researcher, and any experiments or suggestions referred to in these chapters are designed solely for him. Any reader should not attempt, recreate, replicate, or explore them.

Why Research Peptides?

- Research peptides come from a research compounding pharmacy

- They are made for research purposes and not intended for human use

- If a subject decides to do peptide research, it is essential to get from a trustworthy research pharmacy and ensure all their products have been tested, with lab work showing.

- Sigma Compounds is my go-to peptide research pharmacy

- I like using research peptides since they offer a much wider variety of peptides, are much more affordable, and allow me to take my research into my own hands

Figuring Out Which Peptides to Research

Step 1 - Determine Goals, Experience, Health Status & Budget

- Goals

  - Identify the top 1-2 main goals for using peptides (burning fat, better sleep, faster recovery, etc..)

  - This will allow the subject to select the peptide/peptides that best fit this.

- Experience

  - What is the subject's experience with peptides?

  - I recommend starting with 1-2 peptides for the first cycle at a moderate dose.

  - I would increase the peptides I am taking and the stacks once I have a few peptide cycles under my research

- Health Status

  - ⌑ This is important to ensure to get the most out of the peptides.

  - ⌑ Consult with a doctor to ensure specific peptides are a good choice.

- Budget

  - ⌑ Peptides are expensive.

  - ⌑ It is important to budget out per cycle, which most cycles last 2-3 months.

  - ⌑ Factor in the lab supplies.

  - ⌑ Think long-term mindset when going about starting/using peptides

Step 2 - Use Resources and Consult a doctor

- Do not blindly go into peptides

- Use this book to educate yourself on peptides

- Enroll in Peptide Optimization Accelerator to get a deeper dive into therapeutic peptides

- Consult a doctor

Step 3 - Plan & Prepare to Maximize Research

- It is essential to have all the lab supplies and peptides before starting

- Caveat: If new to peptides, I recommend buying a small amount first to see how the subjects respond. It would not be wise to buy a complete peptide cycle and figure out the response is not what was expected

- Focus on lifestyle factors to maximize peptide results.

- Consistency is important

Question to keep in mind

- Is the subject comfortable with the lab supplies and knows how to use them?

- Does the subject know how many injections are given a week/day?

- Does the subject know what time of the day each injection should be administered?

- Will the subject be traveling/busy during the cycle?

- Can the subject afford the complete peptide cycle?

Step 4 - General Research Peptide Protocol Cycle

- General Peptide Cycle Outline

  - ¤ Review the peptide cycle research to determine which peptides are best for the goal. Consult a doctor as needed

  - ¤ Pick out the peptides. Start with 1-2 peptides if new at a moderate dose

  - ¤ Buy all lab supplies and peptide supplies. Familiarize with supplies

  - ¤ Prep for the cycle. It is important and to figure out dosing and frequency of each peptide

  - ¤ Run the cycle for 8-12 weeks (for most peptides)

  - ¤ Take 4-8 weeks off (for most peptides). Reflect and see what went well and what did not go well

  - ¤ Repeat the cycle or adjust based on the goals

Lab Supplies

- Cotton Balls https://amzn.to/3qn02o5

  ¤ For cleaning peptide caps and skin

- Rubbing Alcohol - https://amzn.to/3x0XHDd

  ¤ For sterilizing peptide caps and skin

- 3 ml syringe with a needle head - https://amzn.to/3risCeK

  ¤ For reconstitution (adding bacteriostatic water to peptide)

- 31G-.5/16inch needles - https://amzn.to/3ARWv67

  ¤ For injecting

- Needle Trash Can - https://amzn.to/3xoMsov

  ¤ To properly trash used needles

- Plastic Container - https://amzn.to/3qhJdes

  ¤ To store all lab supplies

- Glass Container with Towel https://amzn.to/3esBjfD

  ¤ To store peptides (want to store them in a cold/dark place)

- Pep Calc App - https://pepcalc.app/

  ¤ To help figure out dosing

- Research Grade Peptide https://sigmacompounds.com/

  ¤ To find the highest quality research peptides

How To Set Up A Research Lab

Why This Is Important

- It is essential to stay organized with peptides to get the most results.

- This is to ensure correct dosing and a clean and efficient injecting process.

- It saves time and makes the entire process easier

How To Set Up Lab for Efficiency

- Ideally, to have this all in a place that has a fridge nearby

- Place all lab supplies except peptides and bacteriostatic water in a plastic container in a cabinet

- Place all peptides and bacteriostatic water in a glass container in the fridge

- Have a needle trash can close by

Understanding Pep-Calc

How To Use Pep-Calc

This is the best app that will help determine dosing

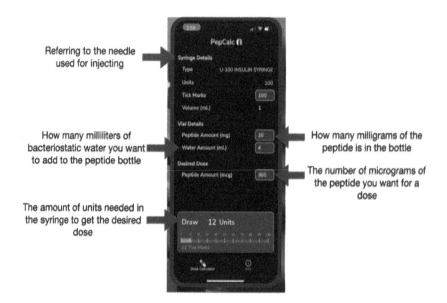

Referring to the needle used for injecting

How many milliliters of bacteriostatic water you want to add to the peptide bottle

How many milligrams of the peptide is in the bottle

The number of micrograms of the peptide you want for a dose

The amount of units needed in the syringe to get the desired dose

How To Reconstitute Peptides

- If buying from a research company, peptides will come in powder and must be reconstituted with bacteriostatic water.

- Most peptide bottles come in 3-4mL bottles, meaning to put up to 3-4mL of bacteriostatic water because more would over-fill it.

Supplies Needed

- 10 mL syringe

- Cotton Balls

- Rubbing Alcohol

- Needle Trash Can

- Bacteriostatic Water

- Peptide

Steps

- Decide how much bacteriostatic water will be using

- Take the cap off the peptide bottle and bacteriostatic water. Clean both areas with rubbing alcohol using a cotton ball

- Take the 3ml syringe and put 2-3ml (depending on how much is being used) of air into the syringe. This will create a reverse pressure

- Inject the 3ml syringe into the bacteriostatic water, turn it upside down, and press the air into it. The water should come into the syringe with little to no effort. Measure from the bottom aspect of the syringe. Turn the bacteriostatic water face up before withdrawing the needle

- Insert the 3ml syringe with bacteriostatic water into the peptide bottle.

- Ideally, angle the bacteriostatic water so it does not directly hit the peptide. And slowly inject the water so as not to damage the peptide

- Once all the bacteriostatic water is in the syringe, slowly withdraw the needle and glide the peptide bottle back and forth between hands to mix the peptide

- Place the syringe and needles into the needle trash can

Measuring Bacteriostatic Water

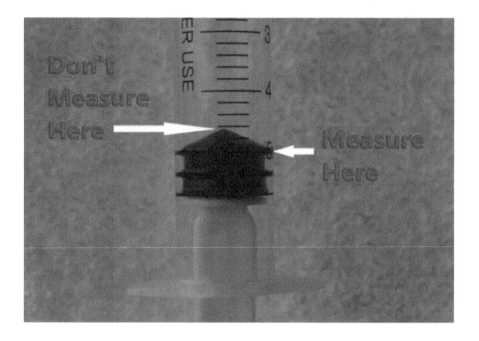

How To Figure Out How Much Bacteriostatic Water To Add?

- Use the app PepCalc to help determine how many units will be needed in the syringe by adding the amount of bacteriostatic water added to the peptide and the desired dose.

- Most peptide vials are 3 mL, meaning more than 3 mL will overflow the vial. I use around 1-3 mL per vial.

- I use 3 mL of bacteriostatic if the peptide is small (MG), and I need a small amount for the dose.

  ⋈ Ex: A 5 MG bottle of Ipamorelin with a desired dose of 200 mcg.

- **1 mL of bacteriostatic water would be -> 4 units** (VERY SMALL and hard to get exactly in a syringe)

- **3 ml of bacteriostatic water would be -> 12 units** (Much easier to get that into a syringe than 4 units)

• I use 1ml of bacteriostatic water if the peptide is large (MG) and I need a large dose.

  ¤ Ex: A 5 MG Bottle of BPC-157 with a desired dose of 500 mcg

    - **3 mL of bacteriostatic water would be -> 30 units** (A lot of fluid to inject, especially if there is multiple peptides being added)

    - **1 ml of bacteriostatic water would be -> 10 units** (Much less fluid and less hassle when injecting)

• I use 2mL of bacteriostatic water for everything else in between. **I often use 2 mL of bacteriostatic water to simplify things.**

How To Prepare a Peptide Injection

Supplies Needed

• 31G-.5/16inch insulin syringe

• Cotton ball

• Peptide

• Rubbing Alcohol

Steps

• Clean peptide bottle with rubbing alcohol

• Insert the insulin syringe into the middle of the peptide bottle

- Tip peptide bottle upside-side down

- Withdraw the desired peptide amount

- Turn the peptide bottle back to facing up right before removing the needle

- Recap insulin syringe

How To Combine Peptides

Combining peptides can be a great way to make unique peptide combinations and make a peptide protocol efficient if multiple peptides are used simultaneously.

This is also a great way to turn multiple injections into just one injection

Start with the peptide that requires the *least amount* and then continue to the peptide that requires the most.

Supplies Needed

- 31G-.5/16inch insulin syringe

- PepCalc App

- Cotton Balls

- Rubbing Alcohol

- Peptides

Steps

- Figure out the dosing of each peptide using Pep calc

- Clean off peptide bottles

- Start with the peptide that requires the least number of units and work up

- Recap the 31G-.5/16inch insulin syringe

How To Inject Peptides

Supplies Needed

- 31-G .5/16inch needle syringe with peptide inside

- Rubbing Alcohol

- Cotton Ball

- Needle Trash Can

Injecting Steps

- Use a cotton ball dipped in rubbing alcohol and clean the surface of the injecting area.

- Withdraw the desired amount of peptide into the 31 Gauge 5/16-inch needle syringe.

- Typical injection locations are the side glute and abdominal region. Find the area with the most adipose (fat)

- Slowly insert the needle. Once the needle is firmly in, slowly release the peptide

- Slowly withdraw and then use a cotton ball dipped in rubbing alcohol to clean the area. Applying deep pressure and massaging the area with the cotton ball can be helpful.

- Dispose of the 31-G 5/16inch needle syringe into the needle trash can

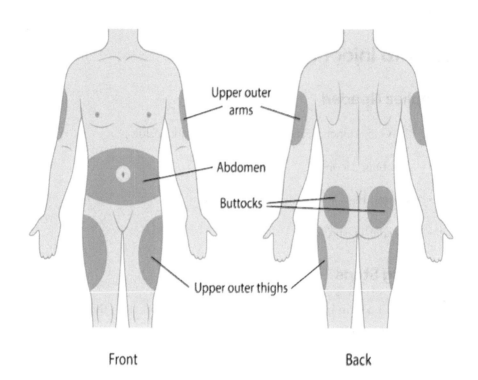

Front   Back

442

18. Master Peptide Therapy

If you are hungry for more and want to dive deeper into therapeutic peptides, I recommend looking into the Peptide Optimization Accelerator. This is a video course that greatly complements this book.

By using the discount code "Peptides" you'll save 30%

Go to this URL to master peptide therapy

https://www.peptide-optimization.com/peptide-optimization-accelerator-course

Thank You

I want to say thank you for taking the time to spend your valuable money and time on this book.

I put a ton of time into creating this, and it was genuine hope that this book could enhance your life

It would mean the world if you could take a moment and leave a review

About The Author

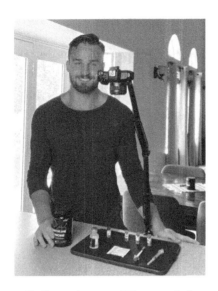

Matthew Farrahi

Matthew's purpose has been helping men (and himself) optimize their lives in a holistic context for the past 10 years. He has dedicated himself to helping men grow physically, emotionally, intellectually, and spiritually stronger, ultimately allowing a man to tap into his most powerful and evolved state.

Growing up, he saw a lack of positive masculine influence worldwide, especially regarding men's health. He struggled on his journey and saw this in many men around him.

He started pursuing this purpose by researching, studying, and experimenting. During this, he was mocked, shamed, and doubted, especially during several of his experiments. However, this did not stop him. He believed in himself, especially the results he saw, and knew what he had could empower men to a new level.

Along his journey, he has been sharing what he has been learning through social media. Through his experiments, he has achieved new heights of health and power.

Matthew's hunger for his purpose has only deepened. He is constantly studying, experimenting, and contemplating men's health to discover new possibilities for men.

Connect With Matthew

News Letter:

Masculine Medicine Research

https://www.manhoodlevelup.com/maxout

Peptide Insights

https://www.peptide-optimization.com/exclusive

YouTube:

@Masculine Medicine Research

https://www.youtube.com/@MasculineMedResearch

@Peptide Insights

https://www.youtube.com/@PeptideInsights

Instagram:

@Matthew_Farrahi

https://www.instagram.com/matthew_farrahi/

@Peptideinsights

https://www.instagram.com/peptideinsights/

@Mmresearch_

https://www.instagram.com/mmresearch_/

Rumble:

@Masculine Medicine Research

https://rumble.com/c/c-2292572

@Peptide Insights

https://rumble.com/c/c-5730776

Twitter - X:

@MasculineMed

https://twitter.com/MasculineMed

@PeptideInsights

https://twitter.com/peptideinsights

Research Peptide Sourcing

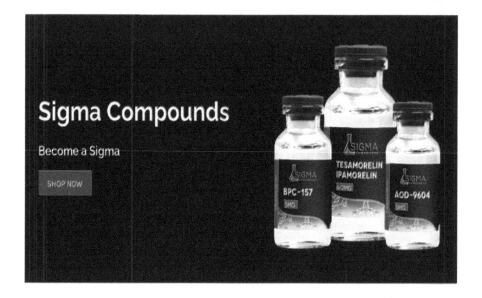

Sigma Compounds Peptides

https://sigmacompounds.com/

Sigma Compounds Peptides offers the most premium peptide experience and is my most trusted source for buying research peptides. They offer the highest quality research peptides by getting

Disclaimer:

Any products for sale or promotion on www.sigmacompounds.com are not for animal or human consumption in any manner, whether directly or indirectly, and are intended solely and exclusively for laboratory research purposes. By using this website, you understand and agree that none of the products for sale or promotion on www.sigmacompounds.com are intended to diagnose, treat, cure, alleviate, or prevent any disease or medical condition and that no claim or warranty is made to that effect.

Bibliography

5-Amin-1-MQ

Kim YB, Peroni OD, Aschenbach WG, Minokoshi Y, Kotani K, Zisman A, Kahn CR, Goodyear LJ, Kahn BB. Muscle-specific deletion of the Glut4 glucose transporter alters multiple regulatory steps in glycogen metabolism. Mol Cell Biol. 2005 Nov;25(21):9713-23. doi: 10.1128/MCB.25.21.9713-9723.2005. PMID: 16227617; PMCID: PMC1265843.

Carvalho E, Kotani K, Peroni OD, Kahn BB. Adipose-specific overexpression of GLUT4 reverses insulin resistance and diabetes in mice lacking GLUT4 selectively in muscle. Am J Physiol Endocrinol Metab. 2005 Oct;289(4):E551-61. doi: 10.1152/ajpendo.00116.2005. Epub 2005 May 31. PMID: 15928024.

Neelakantan H, Vance V, Wetzel MD, Wang HL, McHardy SF, Finnerty CC, Hommel JD, Watowich SJ. Selective and membrane-permeable small molecule inhibitors of nicotinamide N-methyltransferase reverse high fat diet-induced obesity in mice. Biochem Pharmacol. 2018 Jan;147:141-152. doi: 10.1016/j.bcp.2017.11.007. Epub 2017 Nov 15. PMID: 29155147; PMCID: PMC5826726.

Ryu D, Zhang H, Ropelle ER, Sorrentino V, Mázala DA, Mouchiroud L, Marshall PL, Campbell MD, Ali AS, Knowels GM, Bellemin S, Iyer SR, Wang X, Gariani K, Sauve AA, Cantó C, Conley KE, Walter L, Lovering RM, Chin ER, Jasmin BJ, Marcinek DJ, Menzies KJ, Auwerx J. NAD+ repletion improves muscle function in muscular dystrophy and counters global PARylation. Sci Transl Med. 2016 Oct 19;8(361):361ra139. doi: 10.1126/scitranslmed.aaf5504. PMID: 27798264; PMCID: PMC5535761.

SS-31

Szeto HH, Liu S, Soong Y, Wu D, Darrah SF, Cheng FY, Zhao Z, Ganger M, Tow CY, Seshan SV. Mitochondria-targeted peptide accelerates ATP recovery and reduces ischemic kidney injury. J Am Soc Nephrol. 2011 Jun;22(6):1041-52. doi: 10.1681/ASN.2010080808. Epub 2011 May 5. PMID: 21546574; PMCID: PMC3103724.

Siegel MP, Kruse SE, Percival JM, Goh J, White CC, Hopkins HC, Kavanagh TJ, Szeto HH, Rabinovitch PS, Marcinek DJ. Mitochondrial-targeted peptide rapidly improves mitochondrial energetics and skeletal muscle performance in aged mice. Aging Cell. 2013 Oct;12(5):763-71. doi: 10.1111/acel.12102. Epub 2013 Jun 11. PMID: 23692570; PMCID: PMC3772966.

Birk AV, Liu S, Soong Y, Mills W, Singh P, Warren JD, Seshan SV, Pardee JD, Szeto HH. The mitochondrial-targeted compound SS-31 re-energizes ischemic mitochondria by interacting with cardiolipin. J Am Soc Nephrol. 2013 Jul;24(8):1250-61. doi: 10.1681/ASN.2012121216. Epub 2013 Jul 11. PMID: 23813215; PMCID: PMC3736700.

Sabbah HN, Gupta RC, Kohli S, Wang M, Hachem S, Zhang K. Chronic Therapy With Elamipretide (MTP-131), a Novel Mitochondria-Targeting Peptide, Improves Left Ventricular and Mitochondrial Function in Dogs With Advanced Heart Failure. Circ Heart Fail. 2016 Feb;9(2):e002206. doi: 10.1161/CIRCHEARTFAILURE.115.002206. PMID: 26839394; PMCID: PMC4743543.

MK-677

Nass R, Pezzoli SS, Oliveri MC, Patrie JT, Harrell FE Jr, Clasey JL, Heymsfield SB, Bach MA, Vance ML, Thorner MO. Effects of an oral ghrelin mimetic on body composition and clinical outcomes in healthy older adults: a randomized trial. Ann Intern Med. 2008 Nov 4;149(9):601-11. doi:

10.7326/0003-4819-149-9-200811040-00003. PMID: 18981485; PMCID: PMC2757071.

Ney DM. Effects of insulin-like growth factor-I and growth hormone in models of parenteral nutrition. JPEN J Parenter Enteral Nutr. 1999 Nov-Dec;23(6 Suppl):S184-9. doi: 10.1177/014860719902300603. PMID: 10571453.

Adunsky A, Chandler J, Heyden N, Lutkiewicz J, Scott BB, Berd Y, Liu N, Papanicolaou DA. MK-0677 (ibutamoren mesylate) for the treatment of patients recovering from hip fracture: a multicenter, randomized, placebo-controlled phase IIb study. Arch Gerontol Geriatr. 2011 Sep-Oct;53(2):183-9. doi: 10.1016/j.archger.2010.10.004. Epub 2010 Nov 9. PMID: 21067829.

Sevigny JJ, Ryan JM, van Dyck CH, Peng Y, Lines CR, Nessly ML; MK-677 Protocol 30 Study Group. Growth hormone secretagogue MK-677: no clinical effect on AD progression in a randomized trial. Neurology. 2008 Nov 18;71(21):1702-8. doi: 10.1212/01.wnl.0000335163.88054.e7. PMID: 19015485.

FGL(L)

Asua, D., Bougamra, G., Calleja-Felipe, M., Morales, M., & Knafo, S. (2018, February 1). Peptides acting as cognitive enhancers. Neuroscience, 370, 81–87. doi:10.1016/j.neuroscience.2017.10.002

Barco, A., & Knafo, S. (2018, February). Editorial on the Special Issue: Molecules and Cognition. Neuroscience 370,1–3.doi:10.1016/j.neuroscience.2017.11.003 Cognitive boost to brain connections. (2012 February 29). Nature 483(7387), 9. doi:10.1038/483009c

Knafo, S., Venero, C., Sánchez-Puelles C., Pereda-Peréz, I., Franco A., . . . Esteban, J. (2012, February 21). Facilitation of AMPA Receptor Synaptic Delivery as a Molecular Mechanism for Cognitive Enhancement. PLoS Biology 10(2): e1001262. doi:10.1371/journal.pbio.1001262

Cerebrolysin

Gauthier S, Proaño JV, Jia J, Froelich L, Vester JC, Doppler E. Cerebrolysin in mild-to-moderate Alzheimer's disease: a meta-analysis of randomized controlled clinical trials. Dement Geriatr Cogn Disord. 2015;39(5 6):332 47. doi: 10.1159/000377672. Epub 2015 Mar 26. PMID: 25832905.

Masliah E, Armasolo F, Veinbergs I, Mallory M, Samuel W. Cerebrolysin ameliorates performance deficits, and neuronal damage in apolipoprotein E-deficient mice. Pharmacol Biochem Behav. 1999 Feb;62(2):239-45. doi: 10.1016/s0091-3057(98)00144-0. PMID: 9972690.

Rockenstein E, Torrance M, Mante M, Adame A, Paulino A, Rose JB, Crews L, Moessler H, Masliah E. Cerebrolysin decreases amyloid-beta production by regulating amyloid protein precursor maturation in a transgenic model of Alzheimer's disease. J Neurosci Res. 2006 May 15;83(7):1252-61. doi: 10.1002/jnr.20818. PMID: 16511867.

Ruether E, Husmann R, Kinzler E, Diabl E, Klingler D, Spatt J, Ritter R, Schmidt R, Taneri Z, Winterer W, Koper D, Kasper S, Rainer M, Moessler H. A 28-week, double-blind, placebo-controlled study with Cerebrolysin in patients with mild to moderate Alzheimer's disease. Int Clin Psychopharmacol. 2001 Sep;16(5):253-63. doi: 10.1097/00004850-200109000-00002. Erratum in: Int Clin Psychopharmacol 2001 Nov;16(6):372. PMID: 11552768.

AOD-9604

Ng, F. M., Sun, J., Sharma, L., Libinaka, R., Jiang, W. J., & Gianello, R. (2000). Metabolic studies of a synthetic lipolytic domain (AOD 9604) of human growth hormone. Hormone research, 53(6), 274–278. https://doi.org/10.1159/000053183

Cox, H. D., Smeal, S. J., Hughes, C. M., Cox, J. E., & Eichner, D. (2015). Detection and in vitro metabolism of AOD 9604. Drug testing and analysis, 7(1), 31–38. https://doi.org/10.1002/dta.1715

Ng, F. M., Jiang, W. J., Gianello, R., Pitt, S., & Roupas, P. (2000). Molecular and cellular actions of a structural domain of human growth hormone (AOD9401) on lipid metabolism in Zucker fatty rats. Journal of molecular endocrinology, 25(3), 287-298.

Heffernan, M. A., Thorburn, A. W., Fam, B., Summers, R., Conway-Campbell, B., Waters, M. J., & Ng, F. M. (2001). Increase of fat oxidation and weight loss in obese mice caused by chronic treatment with human growth hormone or a modified C-terminal fragment. International journal of obesity and related metabolic disorders : journal of the International Association for the Study of Obesity, 25(10), 1442–1449. https://doi.org/10.1038/sj.ijo.0801740

Ng, F. M., Sun, J., Sharma, L., Libinaka, R., Jiang, W. J., & Gianello, R. (2000). Metabolic studies of a synthetic lipolytic domain (AOD9604) of human growth hormone. Hormone research, 53(6), 274–278. https://doi.org/10.1159/000053183

Kopchick, J. J., Berryman, D. E., Puri, V., Lee, K. Y., & Jorgensen, J. O. (2020). The effects of growth hormone on adipose tissue: old observations, new mechanisms. Nature Reviews Endocrinology, 16(3), 135-146

Heffernan, M., Summers, R. J., Thorburn, A., Ogru, E., Gianello, R., Jiang, W. J., & Ng, F. M. (2001). The Effects of Human GH and Its Lipolytic Fragment (AOD9604) on Lipid Metabolism Following Chronic Treatment in Obese Mice andβ 3-AR Knock-Out Mice. Endocrinology, 142(12), 5182-5189.

Bray, G. A., & Greenway, F. L. (2007). Pharmacological treatment of the overweight patient. Pharmacological reviews, 59(2), 151–184. https://doi.org/10.1124/pr.59.2.2

Heffernan, M., Summers, R. J., Thorburn, A., Ogru, E., Gianello, R., Jiang, W. J., & Ng, F. M. (2001). The effects of human GH and its lipolytic fragment (AOD 9604) on lipid metabolism following chronic treatment in obese mice and beta(3)-AR knock-out mice. Endocrinology, 142(12), 5182–5189. https://doi.org/10.1210/endo.142.12.8522

Kwon, D. R., & Park, G. Y. (2015). Effect of Intra-articular Injection of AOD 9604 with or without Hyaluronic Acid in Rabbit Osteoarthritis Model. Annals of clinical and laboratory science, 45(4), 426–432.

GHK-Cu

Pickart L, Margolina A. Regenerative and Protective Actions of the GHK-Cu Peptide in the Light of the New Gene Data. Int J Mol Sci. 2018 Jul 7;19(7):1987. doi: 10.3390/ijms19071987. PMID: 29986520; PMCID: PMC6073405.

Pickart L, Margolina A. Regenerative and Protective Actions of the GHK-Cu Peptide in the Light of the New Gene Data. Int J Mol Sci. 2018 Jul 7;19(7):1987. doi: 10.3390/ijms19071987. PMID: 29986520; PMCID: PMC6073405.

Pickart L, Vasquez-Soltero JM, Margolina A. The Effect of the Human Peptide GHK on Gene Expression Relevant to Nervous System Function and Cognitive Decline. Brain Sci. 2017 Feb 15;7(2):20. doi: 10.3390/brainsci7020020. PMID: 28212278; PMCID: PMC5332963.

Pickart L, Vasquez-Soltero JM, Margolina A. The human tripeptide GHK-Cu in prevention of oxidative stress and degenerative conditions of aging: implications for cognitive health. Oxid Med Cell Longev. 2012;2012:324832. doi: 10.1155/2012/324832. Epub 2012 May 10. PMID: 22666519; PMCID: PMC3359723.

Zhou XM, Wang GL, Wang XB, Liu L, Zhang Q, Yin Y, Wang QY, Kang J, Hou G. GHK Peptide Inhibits Bleomycin-Induced Pulmonary Fibrosis in Mice by Suppressing TGFβ1/Smad-Mediated Epithelial-to-Mesenchymal Transition. Front Pharmacol. 2017 Dec 12;8:904. doi: 10.3389/fphar.2017.00904. PMID: 29311918; PMCID: PMC5733019.

Park JR, Lee H, Kim SI, Yang SR. The tri-peptide GHK-Cu complex ameliorates lipopolysaccharide-induced acute lung injury in mice. Oncotarget. 2016 Sep 6;7(36):58405-58417. doi: 10.18632/oncotarget.11168. PMID: 27517151; PMCID: PMC5295439.

Sever'yanova LA, Dolgintsev ME. Effects of Tripeptide Gly-His-Lys in Pain-Induced Aggressive-Defensive Behavior in Rats. Bull Exp Biol Med. 2017 Dec;164(2):140-143. doi: 10.1007/s10517-017-3943-3. Epub 2017 Nov 27. PMID: 29181666

Sever'yanova LA, Plotnikov DV. Binding of Glyprolines to L-Arginine Inverts Its Analgesic and Antiagressogenic Effects. Bull Exp Biol Med. 2018 Sep;165(5):621-624. doi: 10.1007/s10517-018-4227-2. Epub 2018 Sep 17. PMID: 30225713

DSIP

Monnier M, Dudler L, Gächter R, Maier PF, Tobler HJ, Schoenenberger GA. The delta sleep inducing peptide (DSIP). Comparative properties of the original and synthetic nonapeptide. Experientia. 1977 Apr 15;33(4):548-52. doi: 10.1007/BF01922266. PMID: 862769.

Koval'zon VM. DSIP: peptid sna ili neizvestnyĭ gormon gipotalamusa [DSIP: the sleep peptide or an unknown hypothalamic hormone?]. Zh Evol Biokhim Fiziol. 1994 Mar-Apr;30(2):310-9. Russian. PMID: 7817664.

Nakagaki K, Ebihara S, Usui S, Honda Y, Takahashi Y, Kato N. [Effects of intraventricular injection of anti-DSIP serum on sleep in rats]. Yakubutsu Seishin Kodo. 1986 Jun;6(2):259-65. Japanese. PMID: 3776352.

Iyer KS, Marks GA, Kastin AJ, McCann SM. Evidence for a role of delta sleep-inducing peptide in slow-wave sleep and sleep-related growth hormone release in the rat. Proc Natl Acad Sci U S A. 1988 May;85(10):3653-6. doi: 10.1073/pnas.85.10.3653. PMID: 3368469; PMCID: PMC280272.

Schneider-Helmert D, Gnirss F, Monnier M, Schenker J, Schoenenberger GA. Acute and delayed effects of DSIP (delta sleep-inducing peptide) on human sleep behavior. Int J Clin Pharmacol Ther Toxicol. 1981 Aug;19(8):341-5. PMID: 6895513.

Larbig W, Gerber WD, Kluck M, Schoenenberger GA. Therapeutic effects of delta-sleep-inducing peptide (DSIP) in patients with chronic, pronounced pain episodes. A clinical pilot study. Eur Neurol. 1984;23(5):372-85. doi: 10.1159/000115716. PMID: 6548970.

Dick P, Grandjean ME, Tissot R. Successful treatment of withdrawal symptoms with delta sleep-inducing peptide, a neuropeptide with potential agonistic activity on opiate receptors. Neuropsychobiology. 1983;10(4):205-8. doi: 10.1159/000118012. PMID: 6328354.

Lesch KP, Widerlöv E, Ekman R, Laux G, Schulte HM, Pfüller H, Beckmann H. Delta sleep-inducing peptide response to human corticotropin-releasing hormone (CRH) in major depressive disorder. Comparison with CRH-induced corticotropin and cortisol secretion. Biol Psychiatry. 1988 Jun;24(2):162-72. doi: 10.1016/0006-3223(88)90271-5. PMID: 2839244.

Khvatova EM, Samartzev VN, Zagoskin PP, Prudchenko IA, Mikhaleva II. Delta sleep inducing peptide (DSIP): effect on respiration activity in rat brain mitochondria and stress protective potency under experimental hypoxia. Peptides. 2003 Feb;24(2):307-11. doi: 10.1016/s0196-9781(03)00040-8. PMID: 12668217.

CJC-1295

Alba M, Fintini D, Sagazio A, Lawrence B, Castaigne JP, Frohman LA, Salvatori R. Once-daily administration of CJC-1295, a long-acting growth hormone-releasing hormone (GHRH) analog, normalizes growth in the GHRH knockout mouse. Am J Physiol Endocrinol Metab. 2006 Dec;291(6):E1290-4. doi: 10.1152/ajpendo.00201.2006. Epub 2006 Jul 5. PMID: 16822960.

Gautam D, Jeon J, Starost MF, Han SJ, Hamdan FF, Cui Y, Parlow AF, Gavrilova O, Szalayova I, Mezey E, Wess J. Neuronal M3 muscarinic acetylcholine receptors are essential for somatotroph proliferation and normal somatic growth. Proc Natl Acad Sci U S A. 2009 Apr 14;106(15):6398-403. doi: 10.1073/pnas.0900977106. Epub 2009 Mar 30. PMID: 19332789; PMCID: PMC2662962.

Teichman SL, Neale A, Lawrence B, Gagnon C, Castaigne JP, Frohman LA. Prolonged stimulation of growth hormone (GH) and insulin-like growth factor I secretion by CJC-1295, a long-acting analog of GH-releasing hormone, in healthy adults. J Clin Endocrinol Metab. 2006 Mar;91(3):799-805. doi: 10.1210/jc.2005-1536. Epub 2005 Dec 13. PMID: 16352683.

Guo S, Li Z, Yan L, Sun Y, Feng Y. GnRH agonist improves pregnancy outcome in mice with induced adenomyosis by restoring endometrial receptivity. Drug Des Devel Ther. 2018 Jun 7;12:1621-1631. doi: 10.2147/DDDT.S162541. PMID: 29922037; PMCID: PMC5995291.

Jetté L, Léger R, Thibaudeau K, Benquet C, Robitaille M, Pellerin I, Paradis V, van Wyk P, Pham K, Bridon DP. Human growth hormone-releasing factor (hGRF)1-29-albumin bioconjugates activate the GRF receptor on the anterior pituitary in rats: identification of CJC-1295 as a long-lasting GRF analog. Endocrinology. 2005 Jul;146(7):3052-8. doi: 10.1210/en.2004-1286. Epub 2005 Apr 7. PMID: 15817669.

BPC-157

Jelovac, N., Sikirić, P., Rucman, R., Petek, M., Perović, D., Konjevoda, P., Marović, A., Seiwerth, S., Grabarević, Z., Sumajstorcić, J., Dodig, G., & Perić, J. (1998). A novel pentadecapeptide, BPC 157, blocks the stereotypy produced acutely by amphetamine and the development of haloperidol-induced supersensitivity to amphetamine. Biological psychiatry, 43(7), 511–519. https://doi.org/10.1016/s0006-3223(97)00277-1

Sikirić, P., Mazul, B., Seiwerth, S., Grabarević, Z., Rucman, R., Petek, M., Jagić, V., Turković, B., Rotkvić, I., Mise, S., Zoricić, I., Jurina, L., Konjevoda, P., Hanzevacki, M., Gjurasin, M., Separović, J., Ljubanović, D., Artuković, B., Bratulić, M., Tisljar, M., … Sumajstorcić, J. (1997). Pentadecapeptide

BPC 157 interactions with adrenergic and dopaminergic systems in mucosal protection in stress. Digestive diseases and sciences, 42(3), 661–671. https://doi.org/10.1023/a:1018880000644

Tkalcević, V. I., Cuzić, S., Brajsa, K., Mildner, B., Bokulić, A., Situm, K., Perović, D., Glojnarić, I., & Parnham, M. J. (2007). Enhancement by PL 14736 of granulation and collagen organization in healing wounds and the potential role of egr-1 expression. European journal of pharmacology, 570(1-3), 212–221. https://doi.org/10.1016/j.ejphar.2007.05.072

Huang, T., Zhang, K., Sun, L., Xue, X., Zhang, C., Shu, Z., Mu, N., Gu, J., Zhang, W., Wang, Y., Zhang, Y., & Zhang, W. (2015). Body protective compound-157 enhances alkali-burn wound healing in vivo and promotes proliferation, migration, and angiogenesis in vitro. Drug design, development and therapy, 9, 2485–2499. https://doi.org/10.2147/DDDT.S82030

Hsieh, M. J., Liu, H. T., Wang, C. N., Huang, H. Y., Lin, Y., Ko, Y. S., Wang, J. S., Chang, V. H., & Pang, J. S. (2017). Therapeutic potential of pro-angiogenic BPC157 is associated with VEGFR2 activation and up-regulation. Journal of molecular medicine (Berlin, Germany), 95(3), 323–333. https://doi.org/10.1007/s00109-016-1488-y

Chang, C. H., Tsai, W. C., Lin, M. S., Hsu, Y. H., & Pang, J. H. (2011). The promoting effect of pentadecapeptide BPC 157 on tendon healing involves tendon outgrowth, cell survival, and cell migration. Journal of applied physiology (Bethesda, Md. : 1985), 110(3), 774–780. https://doi.org/10.1152/japplphysiol.00945.2010

Škrlec, K., Ručman, R., Jarc, E., Sikirić, P., Švajger, U., Petan, T., Perišić Nanut, M., Štrukelj, B., & Berlec, A. (2018). Engineering recombinant Lactococcus lactis as a delivery vehicle for BPC-157 peptide with antioxidant activities. Applied microbiology and biotechnology, 102(23), 10103–10117. https://doi.org/10.1007/s00253-018-9333-6

Krivic, A., Majerovic, M., Jelic, I., Seiwerth, S., & Sikiric, P. (2008). Modulation of early functional recovery of Achilles tendon to bone unit after transection by BPC 157 and methylprednisolone. Inflammation research : official journal of the European Histamine Research Society ... [et al.], 57(5), 205–210. https://doi.org/10.1007/s00011-007-7056-8

Keremi, B., Lohinai, Z., Komora, P., Duhaj, S., Borsi, K., Jobbagy-Ovari, G., Kallo, K., Szekely, A. D., Fazekas, A., Dobo-Nagy, C., Sikiric, P., & Varga, G. (2009). Antiinflammatory effect of BPC 157 on experimental periodontitis in rats. Journal of physiology and pharmacology : an official journal of the Polish Physiological Society, 60 Suppl 7, 115–122.

Tudor, M., Jandric, I., Marovic, A., Gjurasin, M., Perovic, D., Radic, B., Blagaic, A. B., Kolenc, D., Brcic, L., Zarkovic, K., Seiwerth, S., & Sikiric, P. (2010). Traumatic brain injury in mice and pentadecapeptide BPC 157 effect. Regulatory peptides, 160(1-3), 26–32. https://doi.org/10.1016/j.regpep.2009.11.012

Epithalon

Khavinson VKh. Peptides and Ageing. Neuro Endocrinol Lett. 2002;23 Suppl 3:11-144. PMID: 12374906.

Khavinson V, Diomede F, Mironova E, Linkova N, Trofimova S, Trubiani O, Caputi S, Sinjari B. AEDG Peptide (Epitalon) Stimulates Gene Expression and Protein Synthesis during Neurogenesis: Possible Epigenetic Mechanism. Molecules. 2020 Jan 30;25(3):609. doi: 10.3390/molecules25030609. PMID: 32019204; PMCID: PMC7037223.

Yue X, Liu SL, Guo JN, Meng TG, Zhang XR, Li HX, Song CY, Wang ZB, Schatten H, Sun QY, Guo XP. Epitalon protects against post-ovulatory aging-related damage of mouse oocytes in vitro. Aging (Albany NY). 2022 Apr 12;14(7):3191-3202. doi: 10.18632/aging.204007. Epub 2022 Apr 12. PMID: 35413689; PMCID: PMC9037278.

Ilina A, Khavinson V, Linkova N, Petukhov M. Neuroepigenetic Mechanisms of Action of Ultrashort Peptides in Alzheimer's Disease. Int J Mol Sci. 2022

Apr 12;23(8):4259. doi: 10.3390/ijms23084259. PMID: 35457077; PMCID: PMC9032300.

Anisimov VN, Popovich IG, Zabezhinskiĭ MA, Rozenfel'd SV, Khavinson VKh, Semenchenko AV, Iashin AI. [Effect of epitalon and melatonin on life span and spontaneous carcinogenesis in senescence accelerated mice (SAM)]. Vopr Onkol. 2005;51(1):93-8. Russian. PMID: 15909815.

GHRP-2

Phung LT, Inoue H, Nou V, Lee HG, Vega RA, Matsunaga N, Hidaka S, Kuwayama H, Hidari H. The effects of growth hormone-releasing peptide-2 (GHRP-2) on the release of growth hormone and growth performance in swine. Domest Anim Endocrinol. 2000 Apr;18(3):279-91. doi: 10.1016/s0739-7240(00)00050-3. PMID: 10793268.

Titterington JS, Sukhanov S, Higashi Y, Vaughn C, Bowers C, Delafontaine P. Growth hormone-releasing peptide-2 suppresses vascular oxidative stress in ApoE-/- mice but does not reduce atherosclerosis. Endocrinology. 2009 Dec;150(12):5478-87. doi: 10.1210/en.2009-0283. Epub 2009 Oct 9. PMID: 19819949; PMCID: PMC2795722.]

Hu R, Wang Z, Peng Q, Zou H, Wang H, Yu X, Jing X, Wang Y, Cao B, Bao S, Zhang W, Zhao S, Ji H, Kong X, Niu Q. Effects of GHRP-2 and Cysteamine Administration on Growth Performance, Somatotropic Axis Hormone and Muscle Protein Deposition in Yaks (Bos grunniens) with Growth Retardation. PLoS One. 2016 Feb 19;11(2):e0149461. doi: 10.1371/journal.pone.0149461. PMID: 26894743; PMCID: PMC4760683.

Laferrère B, Abraham C, Russell CD, Bowers CY. Growth hormone releasing peptide-2 (GHRP-2), like ghrelin, increases food intake in healthy men. J Clin Endocrinol Metab. 2005 Feb;90(2):611-4. doi: 10.1210/jc.2004-1719. PMID: 15699539; PMCID: PMC2824650.

Chao YN, Sun D, Peng YC, Wu YL. Growth Hormone Releasing Peptide-2 Attenuation of Protein Kinase C-Induced Inflammation in Human Ovarian

Granulosa Cells. Int J Mol Sci. 2016 Aug 19;17(8):1359. doi: 10.3390/ijms17081359. PMID: 27548147; PMCID: PMC5000754.

Zeng P, Li S, Zheng YH, Liu FY, Wang JL, Zhang DL, Wei J. Ghrelin receptor agonist, GHRP-2, produces antinociceptive effects at the supraspinal level via the opioid receptor in mice. Peptides. 2014 May;55:103-9. doi: 10.1016/j.peptides.2014.02.013. Epub 2014 Mar 4. PMID: 24607724.

Sigalos JT, Pastuszak AW. The Safety and Efficacy of Growth Hormone Secretagogues. Sex Med Rev. 2018 Jan;6(1):45-53. doi: 10.1016/j.sxmr.2017.02.004. Epub 2017 Apr 8. PMID: 28400207; PMCID: PMC5632578.

GHRP-6

Subirós N, Pérez-Saad HM, Berlanga JA, Aldana L, García-Illera G, Gibson CL, García-Del-Barco D. Assessment of dose-effect and therapeutic time window in preclinical studies of rhEGF and GHRP-6 coadministration for stroke therapy. Neurol Res. 2016 Mar;38(3):187-95. doi: 10.1179/1743132815Y.0000000089. Epub 2016 Apr 19. PMID: 26311576.

Suda Y, Kuzumaki N, Sone T, Narita M, Tanaka K, Hamada Y, Iwasawa C, Shibasaki M, Maekawa A, Matsuo M, Akamatsu W, Hattori N, Okano H, Narita M. Down-regulation of ghrelin receptors on dopaminergic neurons in the substantia nigra contributes to Parkinson's disease-like motor dysfunction. Mol Brain. 2018 Feb 20;11(1):6. doi: 10.1186/s13041-018-0349-8. PMID: 29458391; PMCID: PMC5819262.

Berlanga J, Cibrian D, Guevara L, Dominguez H, Alba JS, Seralena A, Guillén G, López-Mola E, López-Saura P, Rodriguez A, Perez B, Garcia D, Vispo NS. Growth-hormone-releasing peptide 6 (GHRP6) prevents oxidant cytotoxicity and reduces myocardial necrosis in a model of acute myocardial infarction. Clin Sci (Lond). 2007 Feb;112(4):241-50. doi: 10.1042/CS20060103. PMID: 16989643.

Huang HJ, Zhu XC, Han QQ, Wang YL, Yue N, Wang J, Yu R, Li B, Wu GC, Liu Q, Yu J. Ghrelin alleviates anxiety- and depression-like behaviors induced by chronic unpredictable mild stress in rodents. Behav Brain Res. 2017 May 30;326:33-43. doi: 10.1016/j.bbr.2017.02.040. Epub 2017 Feb 27. PMID: 28245976.

Berlanga-Acosta J, Abreu-Cruz A, Herrera DGB, Mendoza-Marí Y, Rodríguez-Ulloa A, García-Ojalvo A, Falcón-Cama V, Hernández-Bernal F, Beichen Q, Guillén-Nieto G. Synthetic Growth Hormone-Releasing Peptides (GHRPs): A Historical Appraisal of the Evidences Supporting Their Cytoprotective Effects. Clin Med Insights Cardiol. 2017 Mar 2;11:1179546817694558. doi: 10.1177/1179546817694558. PMID: 28469491; PMCID: PMC5392015.

Hexarelin

Ghigo E, Arvat E, Gianotti L, Grottoli S, Rizzi G, Ceda GP, Boghen MF, Deghenghi R, Camanni F. Short-term administration of intranasal or oral Hexarelin, a synthetic hexapeptide, does not desensitize the growth hormone responsiveness in human aging. Eur J Endocrinol. 1996 Oct;135(4):407-12. doi: 10.1530/eje.0.1350407. PMID: 8921821.

Bresciani E, Rizzi L, Coco S, Molteni L, Meanti R, Locatelli V, Torsello A. Growth Hormone Secretagogues and the Regulation of Calcium Signaling in Muscle. Int J Mol Sci. 2019 Sep 5;20(18):4361. doi: 10.3390/ijms20184361. PMID: 31491959; PMCID: PMC6769538.

Mao Y, Tokudome T, Kishimoto I. The cardiovascular action of hexarelin. J Geriatr Cardiol. 2014 Sep;11(3):253-8. doi: 10.11909/j.issn.1671-5411.2014.03.007. PMID: 25278975; PMCID: PMC4178518.

McDonald H, Peart J, Kurniawan N, Galloway G, Royce S, Samuel CS, Chen C. Hexarelin treatment preserves myocardial function and reduces cardiac fibrosis in a mouse model of acute myocardial infarction. Physiol Rep. 2018 May;6(9):e13699. doi: 10.14814/phy2.13699. PMID: 29756411; PMCID: PMC5949285.

Mosa RM, Zhang Z, Shao R, Deng C, Chen J, Chen C. Implications of ghrelin and hexarelin in diabetes and diabetes-associated heart diseases. Endocrine. 2015 Jun;49(2):307-23. doi: 10.1007/s12020-015-0531-z. Epub 2015 Feb 4. PMID: 25645463.

Mosa R, Huang L, Wu Y, Fung C, Mallawakankanamalage O, LeRoith D, Chen C. Hexarelin, a Growth Hormone Secretagogue, Improves Lipid Metabolic Aberrations in Nonobese Insulin-Resistant Male MKR Mice. Endocrinology. 2017 Oct 1;158(10):3174-3187. doi: 10.1210/en.2017-00168. PMID: 28977588; PMCID: PMC5659698.

Imbimbo BP, Mant T, Edwards M, Amin D, Dalton N, Boutignon F, Lenaerts V, Wüthrich P, Deghenghi R. Growth hormone-releasing activity of hexarelin in humans. A dose-response study. Eur J Clin Pharmacol. 1994;46(5):421-5. doi: 10.1007/BF00191904. PMID: 7957536.

IGF-1 LR3

Assefa B, Mahmoud AM, Pfeiffer AFH, Birkenfeld AL, Spranger J, Arafat AM. Insulin-Like Growth Factor (IGF) Binding Protein-2, Independently of IGF-1, Induces GLUT-4 Translocation and Glucose Uptake in 3T3-L1 Adipocytes. Oxid Med Cell Longev. 2017;2017:3035184. doi: 10.1155/2017/3035184. Epub 2017 Dec 20. PMID: 29422987; PMCID: PMC5750484.

Tomas FM, Knowles SE, Owens PC, Chandler CS, Francis GL, Read LC, Ballard FJ. Insulin-like growth factor-I (IGF-I) and especially IGF-I variants are anabolic in dexamethasone-treated rats. Biochem J. 1992 Feb 15;282 (Pt 1)(Pt 1):91-7. doi: 10.1042/bj2820091. PMID: 1371669; PMCID: PMC1130894.

Li N, Yang Q, Walker RG, Thompson TB, Du M, Rodgers BD. Myostatin Attenuation In Vivo Reduces Adiposity, but Activates Adipogenesis. Endocrinology. 2016 Jan;157(1):282-91. doi: 10.1210/en.2015-1546. Epub 2015 Nov 18. PMID: 26580671; PMCID: PMC4701895.

Bailes J, Soloviev M. Insulin-Like Growth Factor-1 (IGF-1) and Its Monitoring in Medical Diagnostic and in Sports. Biomolecules. 2021 Feb 4;11(2):217. doi: 10.3390/biom11020217. PMID: 33557137; PMCID: PMC7913862.

AsghariHanjani N, Vafa M. The role of IGF-1 in obesity, cardiovascular disease, and cancer. Med J Islam Repub Iran. 2019 Jun 17;33:56. doi: 10.34171/mjiri.33.56. PMID: 31456980; PMCID: PMC6708115.

Philippou A, Barton ER. Optimizing IGF-I for skeletal muscle therapeutics. Growth Horm IGF Res. 2014 Oct;24(5):157-63. doi: 10.1016/j.ghir.2014.06.003. Epub 2014 Jun 19. PMID: 25002025; PMCID: PMC4665094.

Ipamorelin

Raun K, Hansen BS, Johansen NL, Thøgersen H, Madsen K, Ankersen M, Andersen PH. Ipamorelin, the first selective growth hormone secretagogue. Eur J Endocrinol. 1998 Nov;139(5):552-61. doi: 10.1530/eje.0.1390552. PMID: 9849822.

Johansen PB, Nowak J, Skjaerbaek C, Flyvbjerg A, Andreassen TT, Wilken M, Orskov H. Ipamorelin, a new growth-hormone-releasing peptide, induces longitudinal bone growth in rats. Growth Horm IGF Res. 1999 Apr;9(2):106-13. doi: 10.1054/ghir.1999.9998. PMID: 10373343.

Andersen NB, Malmlöf K, Johansen PB, Andreassen TT, Ørtoft G, Oxlund H. The growth hormone secretagogue ipamorelin counteracts glucocorticoid-induced decrease in bone formation of adult rats. Growth Horm IGF Res. 2001 Oct;11(5):266-72. doi: 10.1054/ghir.2001.0239. PMID: 11735244.

Adeghate E, Ponery AS. Mechanism of ipamorelin-evoked insulin release from the pancreas of normal and diabetic rats. Neuro Endocrinol Lett. 2004 Dec;25(6):403-6. PMID: 15665799.

Childs MD, Luyt LG. A Decade's Progress in the Development of Molecular Imaging Agents Targeting the Growth Hormone Secretagogue Receptor. Mol Imaging. 2020 Jan-Dec;19:1536012120952623. doi: 10.1177/1536012120952623. PMID: 33104445; PMCID: PMC8865914.

Greenwood-Van Meerveld B, Tyler K, Mohammadi E, Pietra C. Efficacy of ipamorelin, a ghrelin mimetic, on gastric dysmotility in a rodent model of postoperative ileus. J Exp Pharmacol. 2012 Oct 19;4:149-55. doi: 10.2147/JEP.S35396. PMID: 27186127; PMCID: PMC4863553.

Sigalos JT, Pastuszak AW. The Safety and Efficacy of Growth Hormone Secretagogues. Sex Med Rev. 2018 Jan;6(1):45-53. doi: 10.1016/j.sxmr.2017.02.004. Epub 2017 Apr 8. PMID: 28400207; PMCID: PMC5632578.

LL-37

Gordon YJ, Huang LC, Romanowski EG, Yates KA, Proske RJ, McDermott AM. Human cathelicidin (LL-37), a multifunctional peptide, is expressed by ocular surface epithelia and has potent antibacterial and antiviral activity. Curr Eye Res. 2005 May;30(5):385-94. doi: 10.1080/02713680590934111. PMID: 16020269; PMCID: PMC1497871.

Alalwani SM, Sierigk J, Herr C, Pinkenburg O, Gallo R, Vogelmeier C, Bals R. The antimicrobial peptide LL-37 modulates the inflammatory and host defense response of human neutrophils. Eur J Immunol. 2010 Apr;40(4):1118-26. doi: 10.1002/eji.200939275. PMID: 20140902; PMCID: PMC2908514.

Kahlenberg JM, Kaplan MJ. Little peptide, big effects: the role of LL-37 in inflammation and autoimmune disease. J Immunol. 2013 Nov 15;191(10):4895-901. doi: 10.4049/jimmunol.1302005. PMID: 24185823; PMCID: PMC3836506.

Reinholz M, Ruzicka T, Schauber J. Cathelicidin LL-37: an antimicrobial peptide with a role in inflammatory skin disease. Ann

Dermatol. 2012 May;24(2):126-35. doi: 10.5021/ad.2012.24.2.126. Epub 2012 Apr 26. PMID: 22577261; PMCID: PMC3346901. Golec M. Cathelicidin LL-37: LPS-neutralizing, pleiotropic peptide. Ann Agric Environ Med. 2007;14(1):1-4. PMID: 17655171.

Moreno-Angarita A, Aragón CC, Tobón GJ. Cathelicidin LL-37: A new important molecule in the pathophysiology of systemic lupus erythematosus. J Transl Autoimmun. 2019 Dec 17;3:100029. doi: 10.1016/j.jtauto.2019.100029. PMID: 32743514; PMCID: PMC7388365.

Singh D, Vaughan R, Kao CC. LL-37 peptide enhancement of signal transduction by Toll-like receptor 3 is regulated by pH: identification of a peptide antagonist of LL-37. J Biol Chem. 2014 Oct 3;289(40):27614-24. doi: 10.1074/jbc.M114.582973. Epub 2014 Aug 4. PMID: 25092290; PMCID: PMC4183800.

Piktel E, Niemirowicz K, Wnorowska U, Wątek M, Wollny T, Głuszek K, Góźdź S, Levental I, Bucki R. The Role of Cathelicidin LL-37 in Cancer Development. Arch Immunol Ther Exp (Warsz). 2016 Feb;64(1):33-46. doi: 10.1007/s00005-015-0359-5. Epub 2015 Sep 22. PMID: 26395996; PMCID: PMC4713713.

Melanotan I & II

Wensink D, Wagenmakers MAEM, Langendonk JG. Afamelanotide for prevention of phototoxicity in erythropoietic protoporphyria. Expert Rev Clin Pharmacol. 2021 Feb;14(2):151-160. doi: 10.1080/17512433.2021.1879638. PMID: 33507118.

Koikov L, Starner RJ, Swope VB, Upadhyay P, Hashimoto Y, Freeman KT, Knittel JJ, Haskell-Luevano C, Abdel-Malek ZA. Development of hMC1R Selective Small Agonists for Sunless Tanning and Prevention of Genotoxicity of UV in Melanocytes. J Invest Dermatol. 2021 Jul;141(7):1819-1829. doi: 10.1016/j.jid.2020.11.034. Epub 2021 Feb 18. PMID: 33609553; PMCID: PMC9009400.

Lau JKY, Tian M, Shen Y, Lau SF, Fu WY, Fu AKY, Ip NY. Melanocortin receptor activation alleviates amyloid pathology and glial reactivity in an Alzheimer's disease transgenic mouse model. Sci Rep. 2021 Feb 23;11(1):4359. doi: 10.1038/s41598-021-83932-4. PMID: 33623128; PMCID: PMC7902646.do

Carmo JM, da Silva AA, Wang Z, Fang T, Aberdein N, Perez de Lara CE, Hall JE. Role of the brain melanocortins in blood pressure regulation. Biochim Biophys Acta Mol Basis Dis. 2017 Oct;1863(10 Pt A):2508-2514. doi: 10.1016/j.bbadis.2017.03.003. Epub 2017 Mar 6. PMID: 28274841; PMCID: PMC5587353.

Ahmed TJ, Montero-Melendez T, Perretti M, Pitzalis C. Curbing Inflammation through Endogenous Pathways: Focus on Melanocortin Peptides. Int J Inflam. 2013;2013:985815. doi: 10.1155/2013/985815. Epub 2013 May 7. PMID: 23738228; PMCID: PMC3664505.

Wurtman R. Multiple Sclerosis, Melatonin, and Neurobehavioral Diseases. Front Endocrinol (Lausanne). 2017 Oct 23;8:280. doi: 10.3389/fendo.2017.00280. PMID: 29109699; PMCID: PMC5660121

Sande PH, Dorfman D, Fernandez DC, Chianelli M, Domínguez Rubio AP, Franchi AM, Silberman DM, Rosenstein RE, Sáenz DA. Treatment with melatonin after onset of experimental uveitis attenuates ocular inflammation. Br J Pharmacol. 2014 Dec;171(24):5696-707. doi: 10.1111/bph.12873. PMID: 25131343; PMCID: PMC4290711.

Strader AD, Shi H, Ogawa R, Seeley RJ, Reizes O. The effects of the melanocortin agonist (MT-II) on subcutaneous and visceral adipose tissue in rodents. J Pharmacol Exp Ther. 2007 Sep;322(3):1153-61. doi: 10.1124/jpet.107.123091. Epub 2007 Jun 13. PMID: 17567964.

Mod GRF 1-29

Wehrenberg WB, Ling N. In vivo biological potency of rat and human growth hormone-releasing factor and fragments of human growth hormone-

468

releasing factor. Biochem Biophys Res Commun. 1983 Sep 15;115(2):525-30. doi: 10.1016/s0006-291x(83)80176-4. PMID: 6414471.

Schally AV, Zhang X, Cai R, Hare JM, Granata R, Bartoli M. Actions and Potential Therapeutic Applications of Growth Hormone-Releasing Hormone Agonists. Endocrinology. 2019 Jul 1;160(7):1600-1612. doi: 10.1210/en.2019-00111. PMID: 31070727

Ito T, Igarashi H, Pradhan TK, Hou W, Mantey SA, Taylor JE, Murphy WA, Coy DH, Jensen RT. GI side-effects of a possible therapeutic GRF analogue in monkeys are likely due to VIP receptor agonist activity. Peptides. 2001 Jul;22(7):1139-51. doi: 10.1016/s0196-9781(01)00436-3. PMID: 11445245.

Waelbroeck M, Robberecht P, Coy DH, Camus JC, De Neef P, Christophe J. Interaction of growth hormone-releasing factor (GRF) and 14 GRF analogs with vasoactive intestinal peptide (VIP) receptors of rat pancreas. Discovery of (N-Ac-Tyr1,D-Phe2)-GRF(1-29)-NH2 as a VIP antagonist. Endocrinology. 1985 Jun;116(6):2643-9. doi: 10.1210/endo-116-6-2643. PMID: 2859987.

Valcavi R, Jordan V, Dieguez C, John R, Manicardi E, Portioli I, Rodriguez-Arnao MD, Gomez-Pan A, Hall R, Scanlon MF. Growth hormone responses to GRF 1-29 in patients with primary hypothyroidism before and during replacement therapy with thyroxine. Clin Endocrinol (Oxf). 1986 Jun;24(6):693-8. doi: 10.1111/j.1365-2265.1986.tb01666.x. PMID: 3098458.

Semax

Medvedeva EV, Dmitrieva VG, Povarova OV, et al. The peptide semax affects the expression of genes related to the immune and vascular systems in rat brain focal ischemia: genome-wide transcriptional analysis. BMC Genomics. 2014;15:228. Published 2014 Mar 24. doi:10.1186/1471-2164-15-228.

Gusev EI, Martynov MY, Kostenko EV, Petrova LV, Bobyreva SN. Éffektivnost' semaksa pri lechenii bol'nykh na raznykh stadiiakh ishemicheskogo insul'ta [The efficacy of semax in the tretament of patients at different stages of ischemic stroke]. Zh Nevrol Psikhiatr Im S S Korsakova. 2018;118(3. Vyp. 2):61-68. doi:10.17116/jnevro20181183261-68.

Lebedeva IS, Panikratova YR, Sokolov OY, et al. Effects of Semax on the Default Mode Network of the Brain. Bull Exp Biol Med. 2018;165(5):653-656. doi:10.1007/s10517-018-4234-3.

Mars RB, Neubert FX, Noonan MP, Sallet J, Toni I, Rushworth MF. On the relationship between the "default mode network" and the "social brain". Front Hum Neurosci. 2012;6:189. Published 2012 Jun 21. doi:10.3389/fnhum.2012.00189.

Agapova TIu, Agniullin IaV, Silachev DN, et al. Mol Gen Mikrobiol Virusol. 2008;(3):28-32.Scantlebury MH, Chun KC, Ma SC, Rho JM, Kim DY. Adrenocorticotropic hormone protects learning and memory function in epileptic Kcna1-null mice. Neurosci Lett. 2017;645:14-18. doi:10.1016/j.neulet.2017.02.069

Deltheil T, Guiard BP, Cerdan J, et al. Behavioral and serotonergic consequences of decreasing or increasing hippocampus brain-derived neurotrophic factor protein levels in mice. Neuropharmacology. 2008;55(6):1006-1014. doi:10.1016/j.neuropharm.2008.08.001

PEG-MGF

Sun KT, Cheung KK, Au SWN, Yeung SS, Yeung EW. Overexpression of Mechano-Growth Factor Modulates Inflammatory Cytokine Expression and Macrophage Resolution in Skeletal Muscle Injury. Front Physiol. 2018 Jul 26;9:999. doi: 10.3389/fphys.2018.00999. PMID: 30140235; PMCID: PMC6094977.

Goldspink G. Research on mechano growth factor: its potential for optimising physical training as well as misuse in doping. Br J Sports Med. 2005 Nov;39(11):787-8; discussion 787-8. doi: 10.1136/bjsm.2004.015826. PMID: 16244184; PMCID: PMC1725070.

Carpenter V, Matthews K, Devlin G, Stuart S, Jensen J, Conaglen J, Jeanplong F, Goldspink P, Yang SY, Goldspink G, Bass J, McMahon C. Mechano-growth factor reduces loss of cardiac function in acute myocardial infarction. Heart Lung Circ. 2008 Feb;17(1):33-9. doi: 10.1016/j.hlc.2007.04.013. Epub 2007 Jun 19. PMID: 17581790.

Song Y, Xu K, Yu C, Dong L, Chen P, Lv Y, Chiang MYM, Li L, Liu W, Yang L. The use of mechano growth factor to prevent cartilage degeneration in knee osteoarthritis. J Tissue Eng Regen Med. 2018 Mar;12(3):738-749. doi: 10.1002/term.2493. Epub 2017 Oct 6. PMID: 28599103.

Chen JT, Wang Y, Zhou ZF, Wei KW. [Mechano-growth factor regulated cyclic stretch-induced osteogenic differentiation and MMP-1, MMP-2 expression in human periodontal ligament cells by activating the MEK/ERK1/2 pathway]. Shanghai Kou Qiang Yi Xue. 2019 Feb;28(1):6-12. Chinese. PMID: 31080992.

Tang JJ, Podratz JL, Lange M, Scrable HJ, Jang MH, Windebank AJ. Mechano growth factor, a splice variant of IGF-1, promotes neurogenesis in the aging mouse brain. Mol Brain. 2017 Jul 7;10(1):23. doi: 10.1186/s13041-017-0304-0. PMID: 28683812; PMCID: PMC5501366.

Dluzniewska J, Sarnowska A, Beresewicz M, Johnson I, Srai SK, Ramesh B, Goldspink G, Górecki DC, Zabłocka B. A strong neuroprotective effect of the autonomous C-terminal peptide of IGF-1 Ec (MGF) in brain ischemia. FASEB J. 2005 Nov;19(13):1896-8. doi: 10.1096/fj.05-3786fje. Epub 2005 Sep 6. PMID: 16144956.

PT-141

Rosen RC, Diamond LE, Earle DC, Shadiack AM, Molinoff PB. Evaluation of the safety, pharmacokinetics and pharmacodynamic effects of subcutaneously administered PT-141, a melanocortin receptor agonist, in healthy male subjects and in patients with an inadequate response to Viagra. Int J Impot Res. 2004 Apr;16(2):135-42. doi: 10.1038/sj.ijir.3901200. PMID: 14999221.

Rössler AS, Pfaus JG, Kia HK, Bernabé J, Alexandre L, Giuliano F. The melanocortin agonist, melanotan II, enhances proceptive sexual behaviors in the female rat. Pharmacol Biochem Behav. 2006 Nov;85(3):514-21. doi: 10.1016/j.pbb.2006.09.023. Epub 2006 Nov 20. PMID: 17113634.

Clayton AH, Althof SE, Kingsberg S, DeRogatis LR, Kroll R, Goldstein I, Kaminetsky J, Spana C, Lucas J, Jordan R, Portman DJ. Bremelanotide for female sexual dysfunctions in premenopausal women: a randomized, placebo-controlled dose-finding trial. Womens Health (Lond). 2016 Jun;12(3):325-37. doi: 10.2217/whe-2016-0018. Epub 2016 May 16. PMID: 27181790; PMCID: PMC5384512.

Miller MK, Smith JR, Norman JJ, Clayton AH. Expert opinion on existing and developing drugs to treat female sexual dysfunction. Expert Opin Emerg Drugs. 2018 Sep;23(3):223-230. doi: 10.1080/14728214.2018.1527901. Epub 2018 Oct 11. PMID: 30251897.

Ji HX, Zou YL, Duan JJ, Jia ZR, Li XJ, Wang Z, Li L, Li YW, Liu GY, Tong MQ, Li XY, Zhang GH, Dai XR, He L, Li ZY, Cao C, Yang Y. The synthetic melanocortin (CKPV)2 exerts anti-fungal and anti-inflammatory effects against Candida albicans vaginitis via inducing macrophage M2 polarization. PLoS One. 2013;8(2):e56004. doi: 10.1371/journal.pone.0056004. Epub 2013 Feb 14. PMID: 23457491; PMCID: PMC3573073.

Maresca V, Flori E, Picardo M. Skin phototype: a new perspective. Pigment Cell Melanoma Res. 2015 Jul;28(4):378-89. doi: 10.1111/pcmr.12365. Epub 2015 Apr 11. PMID: 25786343.

Feller L, Khammissa RAG, Kramer B, Altini M, Lemmer J. Basal cell carcinoma, squamous cell carcinoma and melanoma of the head and face. Head Face Med. 2016 Feb 5;12:11. doi: 10.1186/s13005-016-0106-0. PMID: 26850723; PMCID: PMC4744388.

Selank

Volkova A, Shadrina M, Kolomin T, Andreeva L, Limborska S, Myasoedov N, Slominsky P. Selank Administration Affects the Expression of Some Genes Involved in GABAergic Neurotransmission. Front Pharmacol. 2016 Feb 18;7:31. doi: 10.3389/fphar.2016.00031. PMID: 26924987; PMCID: PMC4757669.

Kasian A, Kolomin T, Andreeva L, Bondarenko E, Myasoedov N, Slominsky P, Shadrina M. Peptide Selank Enhances the Effect of Diazepam in Reducing Anxiety in Unpredictable Chronic Mild Stress Conditions in Rats. Behav Neurol. 2017;2017:5091027. doi: 10.1155/2017/5091027. Epub 2017 Feb 9. PMID: 28280289; PMCID: PMC5322660.

Sokolov OY, Meshavkin VK, Kost NV, Zozulya AA. Effects of Selank on behavioral reactions and activities of plasma enkephalin-degrading enzymes in mice with different phenotypes of emotional and stress reactions. Bull Exp Biol Med. 2002 Feb;133(2):133-5. doi: 10.1023/a:1015582302311. PMID: 12432865.

Uchakina ON, Uchakin PN, Miasoedov NF, Andreeva LA, Shcherbenko VE, Mezentseva MV, Gabaeva MV, Sokolov OIu, Zozulia AA, Ershov FI. [Immunomodulatory effects of selank in patients with anxiety-asthenic disorders]. Zh Nevrol Psikhiatr Im S S Korsakova. 2008;108(5):71-5. Russian. PMID: 18577961.

Zozulia AA, Neznamov GG, Siuniakov TS, Kost NV, Gabaeva MV, Sokolov OIu, Serebriakova EV, Siranchieva OA, Andriushenko AV, Telesheva ES, Siuniakov SA, Smulevich AB, Miasoedov NF, Seredenin SB. [Efficacy and possible mechanisms of action of a new peptide anxiolytic selank in the therapy of generalized anxiety disorders and neurasthenia]. Zh Nevrol Psikhiatr Im S S Korsakova. 2008;108(4):38-48. Russian. PMID: 18454096.

Agapova TIu, Agniullin IaV, Silachev DN, Shadrina MI, Slominskiĭ PA, Shram SI, Limborskaia SA, Miasoedov NF. [Effect of semax on the temporary dynamics of brain-derived neurotrophic factor and nerve growth factor gene expression in the rat hippocampus and frontal cortex]. Mol Gen Mikrobiol Virusol. 2008;(3):28-32. Russian. PMID: 18756821.

Semenova TP, Kozlovskiĭ II, Zakharova NM, Kozlovskaia MM. [Experimental optimization of learning and memory processes by selank]. Eksp Klin Farmakol. 2010 Aug;73(8):2-5. Russian. PMID: 20919548.

Semenova TP, Kozlovskaya MM, Zakharova NM, Kozlovskii II, Zuikov AV. Effect of selank on cognitive processes after damage inflicted to the cerebral catecholamine system during early ontogeny. Bull Exp Biol Med. 2007 Nov;144(5):689-91. doi: 10.1007/s10517-007-0406-2. PMID: 18683497

Sermorelin

Bagno LL, Kanashiro-Takeuchi RM, Suncion VY, et al. Growth hormone-releasing hormone agonists reduce myocardial infarct scar in swine with subacute ischemic cardiomyopathy. J Am Heart Assoc. 2015;4(4):e001464. Published 2015 Mar 31. doi:10.1161/JAHA.114.001464.

Kanashiro-Takeuchi RM, Szalontay L, Schally AV, et al. New therapeutic approach to heart failure due to myocardial infarction based on targeting growth hormone-releasing hormone receptor. Oncotarget. 2015;6(12):9728-9739. doi:10.18632/oncotarget.3303.

Tang S, Luo Z, Qiu X, et al. Interactions between GHRH and GABAARs in the brains of patients with epilepsy and in animal models of epilepsy. Sci Rep. 2017;7(1):18110. Published 2017 Dec 22. doi:10.1038/s41598-017-18416-5.

Shepherd BS, Johnson JK, Silverstein JT, et al. Endocrine and orexigenic actions of growth hormone secretagogues in rainbow trout (Oncorhynchus mykiss). Comp Biochem Physiol A Mol Integr Physiol. 2007;146(3):390-399. doi:10.1016/j.cbpa.2006.11.004.

Walker RF. Sermorelin: a better approach to management of adult-onset growth hormone insufficiency?. Clin Interv Aging. 2006;1(4):307-308. doi:10.2147/ciia.2006.1.4.307.

Wahid ST, Marbach P, Stolz B, Miller M, James RA, Ball SG. Partial tachyphylaxis to somatostatin (SST) analogues in a patient with acromegaly: the role of SST receptor desensitisation and circulating antibodies to SST analogues. Eur J Endocrinol. 2002;146(3):295-302. doi:10.1530/cjc.0.1460295.

TB-500

Ho, E. N., Kwok, W. H., Lau, M. Y., Wong, A. S., Wan, T. S., Lam, K. K., Schiff, P. J., & Stewart, B. D. (2012). Doping control analysis of TB-500, a synthetic version of an active region of thymosin β☐, in equine urine and plasma by liquid chromatography-mass spectrometry. Journal of chromatography. A, 1265, 57–69. doi:10.1016/j.chroma.2012.09.043.

Kim JH, Lim IR, Park CY, et al. Thymosin β4-Enhancing Therapeutic Efficacy of Human Adipose-Derived Stem Cells in Mouse Ischemic Hindlimb Model. Int J Mol Sci. 2020;21(6):2166. Published 2020 Mar 21. doi:10.3390/ijms21062166.

Goldstein, A. L., Hannappel, E., Sosne, G., & Kleinman, H. K. (2012). Thymosin β4: a multi-functional regenerative peptide. Basic properties and clinical applications. Expert opinion on biological therapy, 12(1), 37–51. doi:10.1517/14712598.2012.634793.

Ehrlich, H. P., & Hazard, S. W., 3rd (2010). Thymosin beta4 enhances repair by organizing connective tissue and preventing the appearance of myofibroblasts. Annals of the New York Academy of Sciences, 1194, 118–124. doi:10.1111/j.1749-6632.2010.05483.x.

Spurney CF, Cha HJ, Sali A, et al. Evaluation of skeletal and cardiac muscle function after chronic administration of thymosin beta-4 in the dystrophin deficient mouse. PLoS One. 2010;5(1):e8976. Published 2010 Jan 29. doi:10.1371/journal.pone.0008976.

Tesamorelin

Rochira, V., & Guaraldi, G. (2017). Growth hormone deficiency and human immunodeficiency virus. Best practice & research. Clinical endocrinology & metabolism, 31(1), 91–111. doi:10.1016/j.beem.2017.02.006.

Falutz, J., Allas, S., Blot, K., Potvin, D., Kotler, D., Somero, M., Berger, D., Brown, S., Richmond, G., Fessel, J., Turner, R., & Grinspoon, S. (2007). Metabolic effects of a growth hormone-releasing factor in patients with HIV. The New England journal of medicine, 357(23), 2359–2370. doi:10.1056/NEJMoa072375.

Stanley, T. L., Falutz, J., Marsolais, C., Morin, J., Soulban, G., Mamputu, J. C., Assaad, H., Turner, R., & Grinspoon, S. K. (2012). Reduction in visceral adiposity is associated with an improved metabolic profile in HIV-infected patients receiving tesamorelin. Clinical infectious diseases : an official publication of the Infectious Diseases Society of America, 54(11), 1642–1651. doi:10.1093/cid/cis251.

Mangili, A., Falutz, J., Mamputu, J. C., Stepanians, M., & Hayward, B. (2015). Predictors of Treatment Response to Tesamorelin, a Growth Hormone-Releasing Factor Analog, in HIV-Infected Patients with Excess Abdominal Fat. PloS one, 10(10), e0140358. doi:10.1371/journal.pone.0140358.

Tuffaha, S. H., Singh, P., Budihardjo, J. D., Means, K. R., Higgins, J. P., Shores, J. T., Salvatori, R., Höke, A., Lee, W. P., & Brandacher, G. (2016). Therapeutic augmentation of the growth hormone axis to improve outcomes following peripheral nerve injury. Expert opinion on therapeutic targets, 20(10), 1259–1265. doi:10.1080/14728222.2016.1188079.

Friedman, S. D., Baker, L. D., Borson, S., Jensen, J. E., Barsness, S. M., Craft, S., Merriam, G. R., Otto, R. K., Novotny, E. J., & Vitiello, M. V. (2013). Growth hormone-releasing hormone effects on brain γ-aminobutyric acid levels in mild cognitive impairment and healthy aging. JAMA neurology, 70(7), 883–890. doi:10.1001/jamaneurol.2013.1425.

Thymosin Alpha 1

King R, Tuthill C. Immune Modulation with Thymosin Alpha 1 Treatment. Vitam Horm. 2016;102:151-78. doi: 10.1016/bs.vh.2016.04.003. Epub 2016 May 24. PMID. 27450734.

Pei F, Guan X, Wu J. Thymosin alpha 1 treatment for patients with sepsis. Expert Opin Biol Ther. 2018 Jul;18(sup1):71-76. doi: 10.1080/14712598.2018.1484104. PMID: 30063866.

Wang G, He F, Xu Y, Zhang Y, Wang X, Zhou C, Huang Y, Zou J. Immunopotentiator Thymosin Alpha-1 Promotes Neurogenesis and Cognition in the Developing Mouse via a Systemic Th1 Bias. Neurosci Bull. 2017 Dec;33(6):675-684. doi: 10.1007/s12264-017-0162-x. Epub 2017 Aug 5. PMID: 28780644; PMCID: PMC5725380.

Romani L, Bistoni F, Gaziano R, Bozza S, Montagnoli C, Perruccio K, Pitzurra L, Bellocchio S, Velardi A, Rasi G, Di Francesco P, Garaci E. Thymosin alpha 1 activates dendritic cells for antifungal Th1 resistance through toll-like receptor signaling. Blood. 2004 Jun 1;103(11):4232-9. doi: 10.1182/blood-2003-11-4036. Epub 2004 Feb 24. PMID: 14982877.

Goldstein AL, Goldstein AL. From lab to bedside: emerging clinical applications of thymosin alpha 1. Expert Opin Biol Ther. 2009 May;9(5):593-608. doi: 10.1517/14712590902911412. PMID: 19392576.

Matteucci C, Grelli S, Balestrieri E, Minutolo A, Argaw-Denboba A, Macchi B, Sinibaldi-Vallebona P, Perno CF, Mastino A, Garaci E. Thymosin alpha 1 and HIV-1: recent advances and future perspectives. Future Microbiol. 2017 Feb;12:141-155. doi: 10.2217/fmb-2016-0125. Epub 2017 Jan 20. PMID: 28106477.

Kharazmi-Khorassani J, Asoodeh A, Tanzadehpanah H. Antioxidant and angiotensin-converting enzyme (ACE) inhibitory activity of thymosin alpha-1 (Thα1) peptide. Bioorg Chem. 2019 Jun;87:743-752. doi: 10.1016/j.bioorg.2019.04.003. Epub 2019 Apr 4. PMID: 30974297.

Kharazmi-Khorassani J, Asoodeh A. Thymosin alpha-1; a natural peptide inhibits cellular proliferation, cell migration, the level of reactive oxygen species and promotes the activity of antioxidant enzymes in human lung epithelial adenocarcinoma cell line (A549). Environ Toxicol. 2019 Aug;34(8):941-949. doi: 10.1002/tox.22765. Epub 2019 May 8. PMID: 31067016.

Day P, Duggal M. Interventions for treating traumatised permanent front teeth: avulsed (knocked out) and replanted. Cochrane Database Syst Rev. 2010 Jan 20;(1):CD006542. doi: 10.1002/14651858.CD006542.pub2. Update in: Cochrane Database Syst Rev. 2019 Feb 05;2:CD006542. PMID: 20091594.

ARA-290

Brines, M., Dunne, A. N., van Velzen, M., Proto, P. L., Ostenson, C. G., Kirk, R. I., Petropoulos, I. N., Javed, S., Malik, R. A., Cerami, A., & Dahan, A. (2015). ARA-290, a nonerythropoietic peptide engineered from erythropoietin, improves metabolic control and neuropathic symptoms in patients with type 2 diabetes. Molecular medicine (Cambridge, Mass.), 20(1), 658–666. https://doi.org/10.2119/molmed.2014.00215

Lois, N., Gardner, E., McFarland, M., Armstrong, D., McNally, C., Lavery, N. J., Campbell, C., Kirk, R. I., Bajorunas, D., Dunne, A., Cerami, A., & Brines, M. (2020). A Phase 2 Clinical Trial on the Use of Cibinetide for the Treatment of Diabetic Macular Edema. Journal of clinical medicine, 9(7), 2225. https://doi.org/10.3390/jcm9072225

O'Leary, O. E., Canning, P., Reid, E., Bertelli, P. M., McKeown, S., Brines, M., Cerami, A., Du, X., Xu, H., Chen, M., Dutton, L., Brazil, D. P., Medina, R. J., & Stitt, A. W. (2019). The vasoreparative potential of endothelial colony-forming cells in the ischemic retina is enhanced by cibinetide, a non-hematopoietic erythropoietin mimetic. Experimental eye research, 182, 144–155. https://doi.org/10.1016/j.exer.2019.03.001

Watanabe, M., Lundgren, T., Saito, Y., Cerami, A., Brines, M., Östenson, C. G., & Kumagai-Braesch, M. (2016). A Nonhematopoietic Erythropoietin Analogue, ARA-290, Inhibits Macrophage Activation and Prevents Damage to Transplanted Islets. Transplantation, 100(3), 554–562. https://doi.org/10.1097/TP.0000000000001026

Huang, B., Jiang, J., Luo, B., Zhu, W., Liu, Y., Wang, Z., & Zhang, Z. (2018). Non-erythropoietic erythropoietin-derived peptide protects mice from systemic lupus erythematosus. Journal of cellular and molecular medicine, 22(7), 3330–3339. https://doi.org/10.1111/jcmm.13608

Zhang, W., Yu, G., & Zhang, M. (2016). ARA-290 relieves pathophysiological pain by targeting TRPV1 channel: Integration between immune system and nociception. Peptides, 76, 73–79. https://doi.org/10.1016/j.peptides.2016.01.003

Humanin

Guo B, Zhai D, Cabezas E, Welsh K, Nouraini S, Satterthwait AC, Reed JC. Humanin peptide suppresses apoptosis by interfering with Bax activation. Nature. 2003 May 22;423(6938):456-61. doi: 10.1038/nature01627. Epub 2003 May 4. PMID: 12732850.

Sousa ME, Farkas MH. Micropeptide. PLoS Genet. 2018 Dec 13;14(12):e1007764. doi: 10.1371/journal.pgen.1007764. PMID: 30543625; PMCID: PMC6292567.

Niikura T. Humanin and Alzheimer's disease: The beginning of a new field. Biochim Biophys Acta Gen Subj. 2022 Jan;1866(1):130024. doi: 10.1016/j.bbagen.2021.130024. Epub 2021 Oct 7. PMID: 34626746.

Xiao J, Kim SJ, Cohen P, Yen K. Humanin: Functional Interfaces with IGF-I. Growth Horm IGF Res. 2016 Aug;29:21-27. doi: 10.1016/j.ghir.2016.03.005. Epub 2016 Apr 7. PMID: 27082450; PMCID: PMC4961574.

Qin Q, Mehta H, Yen K, Navarrete G, Brandhorst S, Wan J, Delrio S, Zhang X, Lerman LO, Cohen P, Lerman A. Chronic treatment with the mitochondrial peptide humanin prevents age-related myocardial fibrosis in mice. Am J Physiol Heart Circ Physiol. 2018 Nov 1;315(5):H1127-H1136. doi: 10.1152/ajpheart.00685.2017. Epub 2018 Jul 13. PMID: 30004252; PMCID: PMC6415743.

Li Z, Sreekumar PG, Peddi S, Hinton DR, Kannan R, MacKay JA. The humanin peptide mediates ELP nanoassembly and protects human retinal pigment epithelial cells from oxidative stress. Nanomedicine. 2020 Feb;24:102111. doi: 10.1016/j.nano.2019.102111. Epub 2019 Oct 23. PMID: 31655204; PMCID: PMC7263384.

Kang N, Kim KW, Shin DM. Humanin suppresses receptor activator of nuclear factor-κB ligand-induced osteoclast differentiation via AMP-activated protein kinase activation. Korean J Physiol Pharmacol. 2019 Sep;23(5):411-417. doi: 10.4196/kjpp.2019.23.5.411. Epub 2019 Aug 26. PMID: 31496878; PMCID: PMC6717796.

Kisspeptin-10

Jayasena CN, Nijher GM, Comninos AN, Abbara A, Januszewki A, Vaal ML, Sriskandarajah L, Murphy KG, Farzad Z, Ghatei MA, Bloom SR, Dhillo WS. The effects of kisspeptin-10 on reproductive hormone release show sexual dimorphism in humans. J Clin Endocrinol Metab. 2011 Dec;96(12):E1963-72. doi: 10.1210/jc.2011-1408. Epub 2011 Oct 5. PMID: 21976724; PMCID: PMC3232613.

George JT, Veldhuis JD, Roseweir AK, Newton CL, Faccenda E, Millar RP, Anderson RA. Kisspeptin-10 is a potent stimulator of LH and increases pulse frequency in men. J Clin Endocrinol Metab. 2011 Aug;96(8):E1228-36. doi: 10.1210/jc.2011-0089. Epub 2011 Jun 1. PMID: 21632807; PMCID: PMC3380939.

Navarro VM. Metabolic regulation of kisspeptin – the link between energy balance and reproduction. Nat Rev Endocrinol. 2020 Aug;16(8):407-420. doi: 10.1038/s41574-020-0363-7. Epub 2020 May 19. PMID: 32427949; PMCID: PMC8852368.

Pazarci P, Kaplan H, Alptekin D, Yilmaz M, Lüleyap U, Singirik E, Pelit A, Kasap H, Yegani A. The effects of daylight exposure on melatonin levels, Kiss1 expression, and melanoma formation in mice. Croat Med J. 2020 Feb 29;61(1):55-61. doi: 10.3325/cmj.2020.61.55. PMID: 32118379; PMCID: PMC7063558.

Comninos AN, Wall MB, Demetriou L, Shah AJ, Clarke SA, Narayanaswamy S, Nesbitt A, Izzi-Engbeaya C, Prague JK, Abbara A, Ratnasabapathy R, Salem V, Nijher GM, Jayasena CN, Tanner M, Bassett P, Mehta A, Rabiner EA, Hönigsperger C, Silva MR, Brandtzaeg OK, Lundanes E, Wilson SR, Brown RC, Thomas SA, Bloom SR, Dhillo WS. Kisspeptin modulates sexual and emotional brain processing in humans. J Clin Invest. 2017 Feb 1;127(2):709-719. doi: 10.1172/JCI89519. Epub 2017 Jan 23. PMID: 28112678; PMCID: PMC5272173.

Shoji I, Hirose T, Mori N, Hiraishi K, Kato I, Shibasaki A, Yamamoto H, Ohba K, Kaneko K, Morimoto R, Satoh F, Kohzuki M, Totsune K, Takahashi K. Expression of kisspeptins and kisspeptin receptor in the kidney of chronic renal failure rats. Peptides. 2010 Oct;31(10):1920-5. doi: 10.1016/j.peptides.2010.07.001. Epub 2010 Jul 17. PMID: 20621140.

Sato K, Shirai R, Hontani M, Shinooka R, Hasegawa A, Kichise T, Yamashita T, Yoshizawa H, Watanabe R, Matsuyama TA, Ishibashi-Ueda H, Koba S, Kobayashi Y, Hirano T, Watanabe T. Potent Vasoconstrictor Kisspeptin-10 Induces Atherosclerotic Plaque Progression and Instability: Reversal by its Receptor GPR54 Antagonist. J Am Heart Assoc. 2017 Apr 14;6(4):e005790. doi: 10.1161/JAHA.117.005790. PMID: 28411243; PMCID: PMC5533042.

VIP

Gonzalez-Rey E, Delgado M. Role of vasoactive intestinal peptide in inflammation and autoimmunity. Curr Opin Investig Drugs. 2005 Nov;6(11):1116-23. PMID: 16312132.

Seo S, Miyake H, Alganabi M, Janssen Lok M, O'Connell JS, Lee C, Li B, Pierro A. Vasoactive intestinal peptide decreases inflammation and tight junction disruption in experimental necrotizing enterocolitis. J Pediatr Surg. 2019 Dec;54(12):2520-2523. doi: 10.1016/j.jpedsurg.2019.08.038. Epub 2019 Aug 30. PMID: 31668399.

Said SI. The vasoactive intestinal peptide gene is a key modulator of pulmonary vascular remodeling and inflammation. Ann N Y Acad Sci. 2008 Nov;1144:148-53. doi: 10.1196/annals.1418.014. PMID: 19076374.

Petkov V, Mosgoeller W, Ziesche R, Raderer M, Stiebellehner L, Vonbank K, Funk GC, Hamilton G, Novotny C, Burian B, Block LH. Vasoactive intestinal peptide as a new drug for treatment of primary pulmonary hypertension. J Clin Invest. 2003 May;111(9):1339-46. doi: 10.1172/JCI17500. PMID: 12727925; PMCID: PMC154449.

Chorny A, Gonzalez-Rey E, Delgado M. Regulation of dendritic cell differentiation by vasoactive intestinal peptide: therapeutic applications on autoimmunity and transplantation. Ann N Y Acad Sci. 2006 Nov;1088:187-94. doi: 10.1196/annals.1366.004. PMID: 17192565.

De Souza FRO, Ribeiro FM, Lima PMD. Implications of VIP and PACAP in Parkinson's Disease: What do we Know So Far? Curr Med Chem. 2021;28(9):1703-1715. doi: 10.2174/0929867327666200320162436. PMID: 32196442.

Mosley RL, Lu Y, Olson KE, Machhi J, Yan W, Namminga KL, Smith JR, Shandler SJ, Gendelman HE. A Synthetic Agonist to Vasoactive Intestinal Peptide Receptor-2 Induces Regulatory T Cell Neuroprotective Activities in Models of Parkinson's Disease. Front Cell Neurosci. 2019 Sep 18;13:421. doi: 10.3389/fncel.2019.00421. PMID: 31619964; PMCID: PMC6759633.

Duggan KA, Hodge G, Chen J, Hunter T. Vasoactive intestinal peptide infusion reverses existing myocardial fibrosis in the rat. Eur J Pharmacol. 2019 Nov 5;862:172629. doi: 10.1016/j.ejphar.2019.172629. Epub 2019 Aug 23. PMID: 31449808.

PE-22-28

Djillani A, Pietri M, Moreno S, Heurteaux C, Mazella J, Borsotto M. Shortened Spadin Analogs Display Better TREK-1 Inhibition, In Vivo Stability and Antidepressant Activity. Front Pharmacol. 2017 Sep 12;8:643. doi: 10.3389/fphar.2017.00643. PMID: 28955242; PMCID: PMC5601071.

A. Djillani, J. Mazella, C. Heurteaux, and M. Borsotto, "Role of TREK-1 in Health and Disease, Focus on the Central Nervous System," Front. Pharmacol., vol. 10, Apr. 2019, doi: 10.3389/fphar.2019.00379.

R. S. Duman, S. Nakagawa, and J. Malberg, "Regulation of adult neurogenesis by antidepressant treatment,"Neuropsychopharmacol. Off. Publ. Am. Coll. Neuropsychopharmacol., vol. 25, no. 6, pp. 836–844, Dec. 2001, doi: 10.1016/S0893-133X(01)00358-X.

H. Moha Ou Maati et al., "Spadin as a new antidepressant: absence of TREK-1-related side effects," Neuropharmacology, vol. 62, no. 1, pp. 278–288, Jan. 2012, doi: 10.1016/j.neuropharm.2011.07.019.

Mazella J, Pétrault O, Lucas G, Deval E, Béraud-Dufour S, Gandin C, El-Yacoubi M, Widmann C, Guyon A, Chevet E, Taouji S, Conductier G, Corinus A, Coppola T, Gobbi G, Nahon JL, Heurteaux C, Borsotto M. Spadin, a sortilin-derived peptide, targeting rodent TREK-1 channels: a new concept in the antidepressant drug design. PLoS Biol. 2010 Apr 13;8(4):e1000355. doi: 10.1371/journal.pbio.1000355. PMID: 20405001; PMCID: PMC2854129.

C. Devader et al., "In vitro and in vivo regulation of synaptogenesis by the novel antidepressant spadin," Br. J. Pharmacol., vol. 172, no. 10, pp. 2604–2617, May 2015, doi: 10.1111/bph.13083.

A. J. Silva, J. H. Kogan, P. W. Frankland, and S. Kida, "CREB and memory," Annu. Rev. Neurosci., vol. 21, pp. 127–148,1998, doi: 10.1146/annurev.neuro.21.1.127.

Q. Lei, X.-Q. Pan, S. Chang, S. B. Malkowicz, T. J. Guzzo, and A. P. Malykhina, "Response of the human detrusor to stretch is regulated by TREK-1, a two-pore-domain (K2P) mechano-gated potassium channel," J. Physiol., vol. 592, no. 14, pp. 3013–3030, Jul. 2014, doi: 10.1113/jphysiol.2014.271718.

Semaglutide

Holst JJ. From the Incretin Concept and the Discovery of GLP-1 to Today's Diabetes Therapy. Front Endocrinol (Lausanne). 2019 Apr 26;10:260. doi: 10.3389/fendo.2019.00260. PMID: 31080438; PMCID: PMC6497767.

Holst JJ. The physiology of glucagon-like peptide 1. Physiol Rev. 2007 Oct;87(4):1409-39. doi: 10.1152/physrev.00034.2006.PMID: 17928588.

Yang Z, Chen M, Carter JD, Nunemaker CS, Garmey JC, Kimble SD, Nadler JL. Combined treatment with lisofylline and exendin-4 reverses autoimmune diabetes. Biochem Biophys Res Commun. 2006 Jun 9;344(3):1017-22. doi: 10.1016/j.bbrc.2006.03.177. Epub 2006 Apr 5. PMID: 16643856

.Tang-Christensen M, Larsen PJ, Thulesen J, Rømer J, Vrang N. The proglucagon-derived peptide, glucagon-like peptide-2, is a neurotransmitter involved in the regulation of food intake. Nat Med. 2000 Jul;6(7):802-7. doi: 10.1038/77535. PMID: 10888930.van

Bloemendaal, L., IJzerman, R. G., Ten Kulve, J. S., Barkhof, F., Konrad, R. J., Drent, M. L., Veltman, D. J., & Diamant, M. (2014). GLP-1 receptor activation modulates appetite- and reward-related brain areas in humans. Diabetes, 63(12), 4186–4196. https://doi.org/10.2337/db14-0849

Ard, J., Fitch, A., Fruh, S., & Herman, L. (2021). Weight Loss and Maintenance Related to the Mechanism of Action of Glucagon-Like Peptide 1 Receptor Agonists. Advances in therapy, 38(6), 2821–2839. https://doi.org/10.1007/s12325-021-01710-0

Friedrichsen, M., Breitschaft, A., Tadayon, S., Wizert, A., & Skovgaard, D. (2021). The effect of semaglutide 2.4 mg once weekly on energy intake, appetite, control of eating, and gastric emptying in adults with obesity. Diabetes, obesity & metabolism, 23(3), 754–762. https://doi.org/10.1111/dom.14280

Gros R, You X, Baggio LL, Kabir MG, Sadi AM, Mungrue IN, Parker TG, Huang Q, Drucker DJ, Husain M. Cardiac function in mice lacking the glucagon-like peptide-1 receptor. Endocrinology. 2003 Jun;144(6):2242-52. doi: 10.1210/en.2003-0007. PMID: 12746281.

During MJ, Cao L, Zuzga DS, Francis JS, Fitzsimons HL, Jiao X, Bland RJ, Klugmann M, Banks WA, Drucker DJ, Haile CN. Glucagon-like peptide-1 receptor is involved in learning and neuroprotection. Nat Med. 2003 Sep;9(9):1173-9. doi: 10.1038/nm919.

Epub 2003 Aug 17. PMID: 12925848.Perry T, Haughey NJ, Mattson MP, Egan JM, Greig NH. Protection and reversal of excitotoxic neuronal damage by glucagon-like peptide-1 and exendin-4. J Pharmacol Exp Ther. 2002 Sep;302(3):881-8. doi: 10.1124/jpet.102.037481. PMID: 12183643.

Perry TA, Greig NH. A new Alzheimer's disease interventive strategy: GLP-1. Curr Drug Targets. 2004 Aug;5(6):565-71. doi: 10.2174/1389450043345245. PMID: 15270203.

Graaf, C.d, Donnelly, D., Wootten, D., Lau, J., Sexton, P. M., Miller, L. J., Ahn, J. M., Liao, J., Fletcher, M. M., Yang, D., Brown, A. J., Zhou, C., Deng, J., & Wang, M. W. (2016). Glucagon-Like Peptide-1 and Its Class B G Protein-Coupled Receptors: A Long March to Therapeutic Successes. Pharmacological reviews, 68(4), 954–1013. https://doi.org/10.1124/pr.115.011395

Shao, S., Nie, M., Chen, C., Chen, X., Zhang, M., Yuan, G., Yu, X., & Yang, Y. (2014). Protective action of liraglutide in beta cells under lipotoxic stress via PI3K/Akt/FoxO1 pathway. Journal of cellular biochemistry, 115(6), 1166–1175. https://doi.org/10.1002/jcb.24763

Hager, M. V., Johnson, L. M., Wootten, D., Sexton, P. M., & Gellman, S. H. (2016). β-Arrestin-Biased Agonists of the GLP-1 Receptor from β-Amino Acid Residue Incorporation into GLP-1 Analogues. Journal of the American

Chemical Society, 138(45), 14970–14979. https://doi.org/10.1021/jacs.6b08323

KPV

Elliott RJ, Szabo M, Wagner MJ, Kemp EH, MacNeil S, Haycock JW. alpha-Melanocyte-stimulating hormone, MSH 11-13 KPV and adrenocorticotropic hormone signalling in human keratinocyte cells. J Invest Dermatol. 2004 Apr;122(4):1010-9. doi: 10.1111/j.0022-202X.2004.22404.x. PMID: 15102092.

Xiao B, Xu Z, Viennois E, Zhang Y, Zhang Z, Zhang M, Han MK, Kang Y, Merlin D. Orally Targeted Delivery of Tripeptide KPV via Hyaluronic Acid-Functionalized Nanoparticles Efficiently Alleviates Ulcerative Colitis. Mol Ther. 2017 Jul 5;25(7):1628-1640. doi: 10.1016/j.ymthe.2016.11.020. Epub 2017 Jan 28. PMID: 28143741; PMCID: PMC5498804.

Zhu W, Ren L, Zhang L, Qiao Q, Farooq MZ, Xu Q. The Potential of Food Protein-Derived Bioactive Peptides against Chronic Intestinal Inflammation. Mediators Inflamm. 2020 Sep 9;2020:6817156. doi: 10.1155/2020/6817156. PMID: 32963495; PMCID: PMC7499337.

Richards DB, Lipton JM. Effect of alpha-MSH 11-13 (lysine-proline-valine) on fever in the rabbit. Peptides. 1984 Jul-Aug;5(4):815-7. doi: 10.1016/0196-9781(84)90027-5. PMID: 6333677.

Dalmasso G, Charrier-Hisamuddin L, Nguyen HT, Yan Y, Sitaraman S, Merlin D. PepT1-mediated tripeptide KPV uptake reduces intestinal inflammation. Gastroenterology. 2008 Jan;134(1):166-78. doi: 10.1053/j.gastro.2007.10.026. Epub 2007 Oct 17. PMID: 18061177; PMCID: PMC2431115.

Song J, Li X, Li J. Emerging evidence for the roles of peptide in hypertrophic scar. Life Sci. 2020 Jan 15;241:117174. doi: 10.1016/j.lfs.2019.117174. Epub 2019 Dec 13. PMID: 31843531.

PTD-DBM

Lee SH, Seo SH, Lee DH, Pi LQ, Lee WS, Choi KY. Targeting of CXXC5 by a Competing Peptide Stimulates Hair Regrowth and Wound-Induced Hair Neogenesis. J Invest Dermatol. 2017 Nov;137(11):2260-2269. doi: 10.1016/j.jid.2017.04.038. Epub 2017 Jun 6. PMID: 28595998.

Kim D, Garza LA. The Negative Regulator CXXC5: Making WNT Look a Little Less Dishevelled. J Invest Dermatol. 2017 Nov;137(11):2248-2250. doi: 10.1016/j.jid.2017.07.826. Epub 2017 Sep 27. PMID: 28967390; PMCID: PMC6399733.

Ryu, Y.C.; Park, J.; Kim, Y.-R.; Choi, S.; Kim, G.-U.; Kim, E.; Hwang, Y.; Kim, H.; Han, G.; Lee, S.-H.; Choi, K.-Y. CXXC5 Mediates DHT-Induced Androgenetic Alopecia via PGD2. Cells 2023, 12, 555. doi: 10.3390/cells12040555.

Lee SH, Kim MY, Kim HY, Lee YM, Kim H, Nam KA, Roh MR, Min do S, Chung KY, Choi KY. The Dishevelled-binding protein CXXC5 negatively regulates cutaneous wound healing. J Exp Med. 2015 Jun 29;212(7):1061-80. doi: 10.1084/jem.20141601. Epub 2015 Jun 8. PMID: 26056233; PMCID: PMC4493411.

Ryu YC, Lee DH, Shim J, Park J, Kim YR, Choi S, Bak SS, Sung YK, Lee SH, Choi KY. KY19382, a novel activator of Wnt/β-catenin signalling, promotes hair regrowth and hair follicle neogenesis. Br J Pharmacol. 2021 Jun;178(12):2533-2546. doi: 10.1111/bph.15438. Epub 2021 May 5. PMID: 33751552; PMCID: PMC8251890.

MOTS-C

Lu H, Wei M, Zhai Y, Li Q, Ye Z, Wang L, Luo W, Chen J, Lu Z. MOTS-c peptide regulates adipose homeostasis to prevent ovariectomy-induced metabolic dysfunction. J Mol Med (Berl). 2019 Apr;97(4):473-485. doi: 10.1007/s00109-018-01738-w. Epub 2019 Feb 6. PMID: 30725119.

Kim KH, Son JM, Benayoun BA, Lee C. The Mitochondrial-Encoded Peptide MOTS-c Translocates to the Nucleus to Regulate Nuclear Gene Expression in Response to Metabolic Stress. Cell Metab. 2018 Sep 4;28(3):516-524. e7. doi: 10.1016/j.cmet.2018.06.008. Epub 2018 Jul 5. PMID: 29983246; PMCID: PMC6185997.

Cataldo LR, Fernández-Verdejo R, Santos JL, Galgani JE. Plasma MOTS-c levels are associated with insulin sensitivity in lean but not in obese individuals. J Investig Med. 2018 Aug;66(6):1019-1022. doi: 10.1136/jim-2017-000681. Epub 2018 Mar 27. PMID: 29593067.

Lee C, Kim KH, Cohen P. MOTS-c: A novel mitochondrial-derived peptide regulating muscle and fat metabolism. Free Radic Biol Med. 2016 Nov;100:182-187. doi: 10.1016/j.freeradbiomed.2016.05.015. Epub 2016 May 20. PMID: 27216708; PMCID: PMC5116416.

Che N, Qiu W, Wang JK, Sun XX, Xu LX, Liu R, Gu L. MOTS-c improves osteoporosis by promoting the synthesis of type I collagen in osteoblasts via TGF-β/SMAD signaling pathway. Eur Rev Med Pharmacol Sci. 2019 Apr;23(8):3183-3189. doi: 10.26355/eurrev_201904_17676. PMID: 31081069.

Hu BT, Chen WZ. MOTS-c improves osteoporosis by promoting osteogenic differentiation of bone marrow mesenchymal stem cells via TGF-β/Smad pathway. Eur Rev Med Pharmacol Sci. 2018 Nov;22(21):7156-7163. doi: 10.26355/eurrev_201811_16247. PMID: 30468456.

Qin Q, Delrio S, Wan J, Jay Widmer R, Cohen P, Lerman LO, Lerman A. Downregulation of circulating MOTS-c levels in patients with coronary endothelial dysfunction. Int J Cardiol. 2018 Mar 1;254:23-27. doi: 10.1016/j.ijcard.2017.12.001. Epub 2017 Dec 6. PMID: 29242099.

Fuku N, Pareja-Galeano H, Zempo H, Alis R, Arai Y, Lucia A, Hirose N. The mitochondrial-derived peptide MOTS-c: a player in exceptional longevity? Aging Cell. 2015 Dec;14(6):921-3. doi: 10.1111/acel.12389. Epub 2015 Aug 20. PMID: 26289118; PMCID: PMC4693465.

Tirzepatide

Ahangarpour, M., Kavianinia, I., Harris, P. W., & Brimble, M. A. (2021). Photo-induced radical thiol–ene chemistry: a versatile toolbox for peptide-based drug design. Chemical Society Reviews, 50(2), 898-944.

Thorens B. (1995). Glucagon-like peptide-1 and control of insulin secretion. Diabete & metabolisme, 21(5), 311–318.

Usdin, T. B., Mezey, E., Button, D. C., Brownstein, M. J., & Bonner, T. I. (1993). Gastric inhibitory polypeptide receptor, a member of the secretin-vasoactive intestinal peptide receptor family, is widely distributed in peripheral organs and the brain. Endocrinology, 133(6), 2861–2870. https://doi.org/10.1210/endo.133.6.8243312

Abu-Hamdah R, Rabiee A, Meneilly GS, Shannon RP, Andersen DK, Elahi D. Clinical review: The extrapancreatic effects of glucagon-like peptide-1 and related peptides. J Clin Endocrinol Metab. 2009 Jun;94(6):1843-52. doi: 10.1210/jc.2008-1296. Epub 2009 Mar 31. PMID: 19336511; PMCID: PMC2690432.

Zaazouee, M. S., Hamdallah, A., Helmy, S. K., Hasabo, E. A., Sayed, A. K., Gbreel, M. I., Elmegeed, A. A., Aladwan, H., Elshanbary, A. A., Abdel-Aziz, W., Elshahawy, I. M., Rabie, S., Elkady, S., Ali, A. S., Ragab, K. M., & Nourelden, A. Z. (2022). Semaglutide for the treatment of type 2 Diabetes Mellitus: A systematic review and network meta-analysis of safety and efficacy outcomes. Diabetes & metabolic syndrome, 16(6), 102511. https://doi.org/10.1016/j.dsx.2022.102511

Thomas, M. K., Nikooienejad, A., Bray, R., Cui, X., Wilson, J., Duffin, K., Milicevic, Z., Haupt, A., & Robins, D. A. (2021). Dual GIP and GLP-1 Receptor Agonist Tirzepatide Improves Beta-cell Function and Insulin Sensitivity in Type 2 Diabetes. The Journal of clinical endocrinology and metabolism, 106(2), 388–396. https://doi.org/10.1210/clinem/dgaa863

Permana, H., Yanto, T. A., & Hariyanto, T. I. (2022). Efficacy and safety of tirzepatide as novel treatment for type 2 diabetes: A systematic review and meta-analysis of randomized clinical trials. Diabetes & metabolic syndrome, 16(11), 102640. https://doi.org/10.1016/j.dsx.2022.102640

Jastreboff, A. M., Aronne, L. J., Ahmad, N. N., Wharton, S., Connery, L., Alves, B., Kiyosue, A., Zhang, S., Liu, B., Bunck, M. C., Stefanski, A., & SURMOUNT-1 Investigators (2022). Tirzepatide Once Weekly for the Treatment of Obesity. The New England journal of medicine, 387(3), 205–216. https://doi.org/10.1056/NEJMoa2206038

Targher G. (2022). Tirzepatide adds hepatoprotection to its armoury. The lancet. Diabetes & endocrinology, 10(6), 374–375. https://doi.org/10.1016/S2213-8587(22)00074-2

Hartman, M. L., Sanyal, A. J., Loomba, R., Wilson, J. M., Nikooienejad, A., Bray, R., Karanikas, C. A., Duffin, K. L., Robins, D. A., & Haupt, A. (2020). Effects of Novel Dual GIP and GLP-1 Receptor Agonist Tirzepatide on Biomarkers of Nonalcoholic Steatohepatitis in Patients With Type 2 Diabetes. Diabetes care, 43(6), 1352–1355. https://doi.org/10.2337/dc19-1892

Gastaldelli, A., Cusi, K., Fernández Landó, L., Bray, R., Brouwers, B., & Rodríguez, Á. (2022). Effect of tirzepatide versus insulin degludec on liver fat content and abdominal adipose tissue in people with type 2 diabetes (SURPASS-3 MRI): a substudy of the randomised, open-label, parallel-group, phase 3 SURPASS-3 trial. The lancet. Diabetes & endocrinology, 10(6), 393–406. https://doi.org/10.1016/S2213-8587(22)00070-5

Solini A. (2022). Tirzepatide and kidney function: an intriguing and promising observation. The lancet. Diabetes & endocrinology, 10(11), 762–763. https://doi.org/10.1016/S2213-8587(22)00258-3

Heerspink, H. J. L., Sattar, N., Pavo, I., Haupt, A., Duffin, K. L., Yang, Z., Wiese, R. J., Tuttle, K. R., & Cherney, D. Z. I. (2022). Effects of tirzepatide versus insulin glargine on kidney outcomes in type 2 diabetes in the SURPASS-4 trial: post-hoc analysis of an open-label, randomised, phase

3 trial. The lancet. Ted r & endocrinology, 10(11), 774–785. https://doi.org/10.1016/S2213-8587(22)00243-1

Wilson, J. M., Nikooienejad, A., Robins, D. A., Roell, W. C., Riesmeyer, J. S., Haupt, A., Duffin, K. L., Taskinen, M. R., & Ruotolo, G. (2020). The dual glucose-dependent insulinotropic peptide and glucagon-like peptide-1 receptor agonist, tirzepatide, improves lipoprotein biomarkers associated with insulin resistance and cardiovascular risk in patients with type 2 diabetes. Diabetes, obesity & metabolism, 22(12), 2451–2459. https://doi.org/10.1111/dom.14174

The End

Made in the USA
Las Vegas, NV
13 September 2024

95245332R00272